EMBEDDIN
PEOPLE'S PART
HEALTH S~~~~~

C000155978

New Approaches

Edited by
Louca-Mai Brady

Foreword by
Kath Evans

First published in Great Britain in 2020 by

Policy Press, an imprint of Bristol University Press
University of Bristol
1-9 Old Park Hill
Bristol
BS2 8BB
UK
t: +44 (0)117 954 5940
e: bup-info@bristol.ac.uk

Details of international sales and distribution partners are available at
policy.bristoluniversitypress.co.uk

British Library Cataloguing in Publication Data
A catalogue record for this book is available from the British Library.

ISBN 978-1-4473-5120-7 paperback
ISBN 978-1-4473-5122-1 ePub
ISBN 978-1-4473-5121-4 ePdf

Cover design: Robin Hawes
Front cover image: Beci Ward

Bristol University Press and Policy Press use environmentally
responsible print partners

Printed in Great Britain by CMP, Poole

This book is dedicated to the memory of Adam Bojelian, whose experiences so powerfully underpin his mother Zoe's contribution to this book in Chapter 2. Adam taught me and so many others that young people's participation in health services is not a matter of life and death, it is more important than that.* It is also dedicated to all the young people who contributed to this book, both directly and indirectly. I hope we have done you justice.

* For more information on Adam's life and poetry:
http://intheblinkofaneyepoemsbyadambojelian.blogspot.com/

Contents

List of boxes, figures and tables

Figures

Tables

Summary

While there is growing awareness of the case for children and young people's participation across the UK public sector and internationally, there is limited evidence on how this apparent commitment to participation and children's rights translates into professional practice and young people's experience of participation in health services. Participation in healthcare tends to be driven by a public involvement and engagement agenda rather than more radical models of participatory practice. Young people's views are still not consistently sought or acknowledged within healthcare settings; they are rarely involved in decision-making processes and often occupy a marginalised position in healthcare encounters. Furthermore, much participation is still controlled by adults. In addition to the piecemeal approach to participation in health services there have also been disparities in the characteristics of young people likely to participate, the types of decisions they are involved in making and the extent to which this participation is meaningful and effective. Drawing on Brady's original research and an edited collection of examples of participation in English health practice, *Embedding Young People's Participation in Health Services: New Approaches* explores how the rhetoric of young people's participation can be translated into practice.

Notes on contributors

Chris Affleck joined Investing in Children in March 2015 having previously worked with children and young people in a range of engagement roles with Local Authorities and VCS Organisations across the North East. He is the Mental Health Lead for the organisation and works very closely with the Clinical Commissioning Groups and colleagues in Public Health to ensure that children and young people have opportunities to shape mental health services in County Durham, based on their lived experience. Some of his projects include: facilitating the Young Adult Support Cafes (YASC); coordinating the County Wide and Locality Children and Young People's Emotional Wellbeing Networks; coordinating the County Durham mental health anti-stigma and discrimination campaign Stamp It Out; and supporting the County Durham Time To Change Hub.

Sammy Ainsworth chairs the Board of Trustees for RAiISE and also acts as a parent representative. She is also the Youth and Family Participation Officer for the National Institute for Health Research Alder Hey Clinical Research Facility, where she facilitates the young person and parent research advisory groups under the umbrella of GenerationR (a national Young Person's Advisory Group). She is also a trustee of Lupus UK, and a board member of the European Network for Children with Arthritis.

Sophie Ainsworth is the Founder and CEO of RAiISE, a young people-led UK charity. She is a young person with lived experience of an invisible illness, which led her to establish RAiISE in 2016, following negative experiences in school. She is also a member of several patient advisory groups, including the National Institute for Health Research INVOLVE Advisory

Group and the North West Lupus UK committee. She also has experience of being involved in research.

Louca-Mai Brady has longstanding interests in children and young people's participation and facilitating their involvement in health and social care policy, practice and research. She is currently Senior Research Fellow at University College London Institute of Ophthalmology, where she supports young people's involvement in eye and vision research and Moorfields paediatric services, alongside work as a freelance researcher, consultant and trainer. Louca-Mai has a background in applied social research in academia and the voluntary and public sectors, including leading the development of children and young people's involvement at the Centre for Public Engagement at Kingston and St George's University, the Disability Rights Commission, and as a senior researcher at the National Children's Bureau Research Centre. This book developed from her doctoral research at the University of the West of England on 'embedding young people's participation in health services and research'.

Chloe Brown became involved with Investing in Children as a young person. She went on to become an Investing in Children Project Worker after graduating from Durham University in 2013 where she studied Education and Psychology. Chloe facilitates several projects and has worked with a wide range of services across the UK to ensure that children and young people are able to have a say and that they are listened to. She has particular experience of working with children and young people in healthcare settings and within nursery and school settings. Her aim and passion it to ensure that every child and young person is able to have a say about all aspects of their lives, no matter how big or small those decisions might be. Chloe and Helen Mulhearn Brown have been responsible for the development of the Investing in Children Type 1 Kidz project for children and young people with type 1 diabetes.

Liam Cairns worked with children, young people and their families for over twenty years, in a variety of social work posts, in different local authorities in Scotland and the north of England, before becoming the Director of Investing in Children when it became operational in 1997. Originally based in County Durham, and resourced by the local authority and the NHS, Investing in Children is an organisation concerned with the human rights of children and young people. In 2013 the organisation became an independent Community Interest Company and now works with partners across the UK and Europe. Investing in Children has developed a range of innovative strategies designed to create opportunities for children and young people to contribute effectively to debate and become active participants in democratic processes. Liam has published a number of articles about the position of children and young people in society, and in particular, how children and young people themselves have contributed directly to the learning that has informed the development of Investing in Children.

Robyn Challinor is a young person with lived experience of invisible illnesses, who was motivated to join several research programmes and advisory groups, including being an early member of GenerationR, now a national and international young people's advisory group for health research. She has since graduated from university with a masters degree and currently works in local government as an Assistant Development Officer.

Marie Clapham is RAiISE's Treasurer and was a Special Educational Needs Co-ordinator and secondary school teacher for 13 years. She is now a content writer and team leader for an educational publishing company. As well as her education background, Marie has lived experience of invisible illnesses, bringing her unique perspective across the health and education sectors.

Kath Evans is a registered general and children's nurse. Kath's career has included clinical, educational, managerial, service improvement and commissioning roles. Kath was Experience of Care Lead for Maternity, Infants, Children and Young People at NHS England where she was committed to ensuring the voices of children, young people, families/carers and maternity service users were heard in their care and in the design, delivery and commissioning of services. A highlight of her time at NHS England was establishing the National NHS Youth Forum, securing the implementation of the Children's and Young People's National Inpatient Survey and achieving an increasing national profile of experience, participation and insight work relating to children and young people. Kath has since returned to clinical practice, joining Barts Health NHS Trust as their Director of Children's Nursing, she is Chair of the Children's Health Clinical Board, works with East London Health and Care Partnership as their Clinical Lead for Children and Young People, and is an Academic Nursing Fellow at City University, UK. Kath is a keen user of social media to engage with children, young people, families/carers as well as professionals regarding child health.

Amy Feltham is a psychologist studying how individuals and society manage health and illness. She has a special interest in shared decision-making, which began when she worked as a young participant at YoungMinds, a UK youth mental health charity. She went on to work as a project engagement worker for Common Room, which aims to improve children and young people's involvement in health and social care services. She has worked with others to develop and deliver support for health professionals, including the model and training for the award-winning MeFirst project and the Open Talk model discussed in this book. She recently moved on from Common Room, and currently works directly with disabled children alongside her research. Her input into this book draws on her lived experience of using children's mental health services along with the knowledge she has gained through her work and research.

Ann Hagell is Research Lead at the Association for Young People's Health, UK. Ann is a chartered psychologist with a specific interest in young people. She has published widely on young people's health and is passionate about improving access to information about young people's health in order to improve policy and practice. She is also Counselling Editor for the Journal of Adolescence, and a member of the World

Health Organisation GAMA (Global Action for Measurement of Adolescent health) Advisory Group.

Felicity Hathway completed a mental health nursing degree in 2017 and now works in a Child and Adolescent Mental Health Service unit as a staff nurse. She has a background of lived experience of mental health services and an enduring interest in children and young people's participation. As a young advisor she was extensively involved in participation with organisations including Barnardos, YoungMinds and the Anna Freud Centre. She has delivered training locally and nationally as well as offering consultation to NHS Employers for official guidance on involving children and young people in the recruitment process. Felicity's contribution to this book emerged from her involvement as a young advisor, alongside other young people with experience of participation in health services, in a project on embedding young people's participation in health services.

Lizzy Horn's interest in young people's involvement in healthcare began from her own experiences of accessing both physiological and psychological services as a teenager. She spent 5 years working with a Barnardos service helping children, young people (CYP) and families have a voice about their care, and the services they accessed, in order to make services more CYP-friendly. This included assessing services, being on interview panels for new staff, helping to shape services, finding user-friendly ways to deliver information and sharing her lived experience with local professionals in order to help them feel more comfortable and confident in supporting CYP's mental health. She has since independently done talks to both young people, school staff, and Special Educational Needs Coordinators in the South West. Lizzy's contribution to this book emerged from her involvement as a young advisor, alongside other young people with experience of participation in health services, in a project on embedding CYP's participation in health services.

Sarah Kendal is a mental health nurse and a Research Fellow at the University of Leeds, UK. Her work focuses on improving mental health and emotional wellbeing outcomes for young people and she has broad-ranging experience of projects in that field. Her research is informed by principles of meaningful engagement of young people and uses participatory strategies and research methods. Sarah has published widely on aspects of nursing and mental health in school, hospital and community settings and digital spaces.

Mike Linney is a consultant paediatrician working on the South Coast of England since 2001 with interests in general and respiratory paediatrics and was previously clinical lead for a regional critical care network. He has been a Senior Officer (Registrar) of the Royal College of Paediatrics and Child Health (RCPCH) since 2017 and RCPCH lead for Children and Young People, supporting the experienced CYP engagement team. He has experience in planning national strategies for paediatric care and national reviews of best practice.

Kate Martin has longstanding interests in involving young people in decisions and issues that affect their lives, driven by her lived experience of being a young carer and of supporting family members with long term mental health difficulties. Kate is now the Lived Experience and Engagement Lead for the Wellcome Trust's Mental Health Priority Area, a global programme to better understand, prevent and address anxiety and depression in young people 14–24. Kate has particular expertise in shared decision-making, coproduction, and the issues children and young people experience when living with disability, health or mental health difficulties. In 2019 Kate completed a PhD at University College London exploring shared decision-making with young people in mental health inpatient units. Kate is also Chair of London Friend, a charity which supports the health and mental health of the LGBT community in and around London.

Joanne McAllister is a registered nurse with over 25 years' experience of working within the NHS. She moved into corporate nursing and specialised in Patient Experience. Her passions lie in improving the Children & Young person's experience in acute & community care based upon her own personal experiences of caring for her daughter who has complex learning disabilities. Currently she is a Head of Patient Experience at Pennine Acute Hospitals NHS Trust which is part of the Northern Care Alliance NHS Group.

Helen Mulhearn joined Investing in Children in 2000 and has been a Co-Director of the organisation since it became a Community Interest Company in 2013. Previously, she had extensive experience working within Durham County Council's Children's Services in a variety of roles since February 1992. Helen qualified as a local youth worker with Durham County Council at the age of 17 and completed her training as a Youth and Community worker in 1991 at the University of Birmingham. All of her professional experience has involved working with children and young people and their families, passionately promoting their right to be heard and influence the world around them. Helen and Chloe Brown have been responsible for the development of the Investing in Children Type 1 Kidz project for children and young people with type 1 diabetes.

Barry Percy-Smith is Professor of Childhood, Youth and Participatory Practice at the University of Huddersfield, UK. He has extensive experience as a participatory action researcher in research, evaluation and development projects with children, young people and practitioners in a wide range of public sector and community contexts. He has undertaken numerous projects concerning the theory and practice of child and youth participation including a cross EU evaluation of children's participation and the EU H2020 PARTISPACE project. He has published widely on these issues including *A Handbook of Children and Young People's Participation: Perspectives from Theory and Practice* (co-edited with Nigel Patrick Thomas, Routledge 2010).

Julia Petty is a children's nurse lecturer at the University of Hertfordshire, UK and leads on a variety of child specific and generic nursing modules for the BSc Honours Nursing degree. She is also an executive member and vice chair of the

UK Neonatal Nurses Association and co-chairs a national UK special interest group in neonatal education / research. She is the UK representative on the Board for the Council of International Neonatal Nurses (COINN), a newborn life support instructor for the UK Resuscitation Council and a coach for the UK Council of Deans Student Leadership programme. Her research interests focus on the parent experience with neonatal and children's healthcare education. She has also been part of a research team that has explored the views of young people within the UK NHS Youth Forum, which led to her co-involvement in this book alongside her colleagues from the University of Hertfordshire.

Zoe Picton-Howell is a tutor of Medical Education at Edinburgh University's Medical School. She has also taught healthcare law and law generally for over a decade. Zoe is a solicitor and has a research interest in both child and equality healthcare law. Zoe has served on numerous national research, guidance and investigation committees related to child health and speaks regularly at academic and healthcare conferences in the UK and abroad. Whilst living in Scotland, Zoe was a trustee and director of the Scottish Alliance for Childrens' Rights, in this capacity, she wrote a paper on disabled children's rights in healthcare in the UK submitted to and cited by the UNCRC committee. Zoe is also a director of the Adam Bojelian Foundation and mum to the late Adam Bojelian who was a multi award winning poet and healthcare advocate.

Jennifer Preston currently has a full-time senior Patient and Public Involvement position at the University of Liverpool, UK based at Alder Hey Children's Hospital in Liverpool. Jenny has worked with the National Institute for Health Research (NIHR) in the UK since 2006, on numerous initiatives and projects. Her main role is to deliver a strategy for the involvement and engagement of young people and families in the design and conduct of paediatric health research in the UK, Europe and internationally.

Emma Rigby is Chief Executive of the Association for Young People's Health, UK. Emma has led AYPH since 2008 working at a national level to improve young people's health. She leads a consortia of youth and young people's health charities and works to champion young people's participation and better understanding of young people's health needs and experiences with Government departments, the NHS and Public Health bodies.

Emily Roberts is now freelance after over 10 years with Barnardo's managing an innovative participation service with NHS children's community services in Bristol and South Gloucestershire. A social worker by background, Emily's passion in children's rights began in her safeguarding social care work. This led her to set up and lead a rights and participation service for and with children in care. Joining Barnardo's Emily advocated for participation with parents and younger children as part of one of the trailblazing Sure Start programmes. Contribution to this book followed Emily putting her service forward to feature as a case study in Louca-Mai Brady's doctoral research on 'embedding young people's participation in health services' where young people NHS and Barnardo's staff worked together to identify and showcase ' what good participation looks like'.

Sheila Roberts is currently Senior Lecturer in Children's Nursing at the University of Hertfordshire, UK where her particular responsibilities are for selection and recruitment as well as being part of the team delivering the pre-registration nursing curriculum to student children's nurses. Sheila is involved in a robust service user involvement project with local children and young people which includes involving the children and young people in selection events, health promotion forums, being 'patients' for practical exams as well as sharing their experiences with the students in the classroom. Prior to moving into education, Sheila trained as a RSCN/RN at the Queen Elizabeth School of Nursing, Birmingham, working primarily at Birmingham Children's hospital before holding a variety of posts within acute paediatric care. Sheila has been involved in an evaluative research study with the NHS England

Youth Forum and it is from this that her contribution to this book has emerged.

Emma Sparrow has been a youth and community development worker since 2002 with interests in child and youth participation within strategic decision making. Since 2005 she has been the Royal College of Paediatrics and Child Health (RCPCH) Children and Young People's Engagement Manager, supporting children, young people and families to be actively involved in shaping health policy and practice. She has experience in volunteer management, children's rights, child and youth participation at a local, national and UK level.

Lindsay Starbuck is Youth Participation Coordinator at the Association for Young People's Health, UK. Lindsay has been a youth participation practitioner for over 20 years. She has worked at AYPH since 2011, focusing specifically on increasing marginalised young people's access to good health. Lindsay is committed to using popular education and rights-based approaches that recognise the assets and agency of young people with lived experience of trauma and discrimination.

Simon Stones is an award-winning patient leader, advocate, speaker and consultant, who was the winner of the first international WEGO Health Award for Patient Healthcare Collaborator. He has undertaken a PhD in applied health research, where he developed a programme specification to enhance the supported self-management of arthritis by children and their families. Simon is an active patient research partner on a large number of national and international research initiatives and is a board member of three other associations alongside RAiISE: the European Network for Children with Arthritis, Fibromyalgia Action UK and the European Network of Fibromyalgia Associations, of which he was elected President in 2019.

Kirsche Walker is a Politics and International Relations student and young member of the Association for Young People's Health (AYPH) Advisory Committee. Kirsche has been an engaged participant in empowering young people from the age of 15. She has been involved in many projects over the past eleven years such as: Be Healthy, Our Voices Too and the Young Research Advisory Panel at the University of Bedfordshire (UoB). Kirsche continues to work with AYPH and the International Centre at the UoB to advocate for the importance of involving young people as participants in research. She is passionate about young people's autonomy, empowerment and how research can benefit them and others. Kirsche is currently focusing on accessible and inclusive education on environmental issues, particularly with working class communities and hard to reach young people.

Jack Welch is a graduate in BA (Hons.) Creative Writing and English. For over five years Jack has worked across a number of diverse voluntary sector organisations in a range of capacities. His work was integral to the Heritage Lottery Funded projects 'Dorset Young Remembers' and 'Walking in their Shoes'. Jack has participated with vInspired, the British Youth Council and the National Council for Voluntary Youth Services. He also produced a report for the Department for Communities and Local Government with a series of recommendations on how young people in social housing can be engaged in their communities. He is currently working as an advocate on learning disabilities with Mencap.

Lisa Whiting is Professional Lead for Children's Nursing at the University of Hertfordshire, UK. Her background is as a nurse who worked within a paediatric critical care setting. Since moving to a university environment, Lisa has been involved in the teaching and assessment of undergraduate and postgraduate students across a range of academic levels, including doctoral studies. Lisa completed a doctorate in 2012, her work used a photo-elicitation approach to gain insight into children's wellbeing; since then, she has led several research projects that have spanned a range of child health issues and that have had a strong focus on the involvement of, and the voice of, children, young people and their families. Other research has had an educational remit and has centred on the enhancement of learning for nurses working within areas of child health and children's nursing. Lisa has published and presented her work in a variety of arenas.

Laura Whitty is one of RAiISE's newest trustees, who has a wealth of experience in administration and management across various sectors, including the NHS, children's services and education. Laura is currently an administrator of the Experimental Arthritis Treatment Centre for Children (EATC4Children), based at the University of Liverpool, UK and Alder Hey Children's Hospital in Liverpool as well as an awards administrator for Vasculitis UK. Laura has lived experience with invisible illness throughout her life and this has given her a passion for improving the lives of children, whether that be through driving awareness, education, safeguarding or medicine.

Barry Williams is currently the External Partnership Manager for the Northern Care Alliance NHS Group, based in the north east sector of Greater Manchester. Barry has fifteen years' experience in the NHS delivering patient experience and engagement programmes of work; supporting nursing, clinical and AHP colleagues to embrace patient engagement, highlight its value, interpret, analyse and draw up actions in response to patient experience metrics. Barry's key strength is in establishing partnerships and networks aligned to shared objective with patient representative groups, and the third sector organisations to embed learning and improvement from patient experience across Northern Care Alliance. Barry and his colleagues were 2016 Nursing Times Awards finalists for engagement with young people at Pennine Acute Hospitals.

Acknowledgements

Thanks to the University of the West of England for funding the studentship which led to this book, supervised by Professors Barry Percy-Smith and David Evans. Particular thanks to Professor Percy-Smith for his support and guidance in the development of this book. Thanks as well to all the contributors and those who assisted them, and to Kath Evans for her invaluable support.

Foreword

Kath Evans

I was reflecting on the importance of children and young people's active participation in their healthcare, along with their broader contribution of participating in service development at a commissioning meeting recently. Around the table sat professionals, all with many letters after their names and years of experience in providing and commissioning of healthcare, yet not one of them was under 25. As is usual in these types of gatherings we got on to the subject of 'so what do children and young people want?' We had plenty of reports to refer to, from HealthWatch colleagues who regularly engage with children and young people about 'what matters most to them', to insights from local Trusts who have youth forums, along with representatives at the table from voluntary organisations who help make connections with relevant population groups, and insights from digital engagement on a variety of social media platforms. Yet it was a colleague who made me think when she referred to some national engagement work with children and young people: "Well, the engagement work has been done, we can use that and push on", she commented. It made me reflect that of course we can use engagement work done by others to inform ongoing service improvement, but if we just do that we haven't really 'got' the real 'magic' of participation and the personal development and other benefits it brings for children and young people.

Healthcare professionals still view participation through the lens of providing beneficial insight to providers of services which will ideally lead to improved experience and outcomes for current and future service users. Yet the benefits of participation are much broader. The fact is participation and meaningful co-production not only benefit health services, there is the additional element that the children and young people who engage in the process flourish and thrive when they are active participants as partners in improvement journeys. The contribution of children and young people benefits not only their physical and mental wellbeing, but that of their peers and families as they convey vital health information that they have been involved in, in meaningful ways. It helps address inequalities by raising aspirations, it connects children and young people with potential role models and offers ideas on possible future careers, such as healthcare scientists, administration support, medics, allied health professionals, nurses, information technology specialists – I could go on, after all there are over 350 different careers in the NHS! The creation of participation and meaningful involvement opportunities is an important contribution to the future NHS workforce.

The challenge for health professionals and policymakers is therefore not only to be passive recipients of engagement work, but to create opportunities for children and young people to be an integral part of local systems, providing them with access to role models, insight into the world of health, and volunteering opportunities so that they actively grow in confidence as their experiences are valued, nurtured and life skills expanded. The challenge for researchers working in the field is to consider how best to work with health professionals, policymakers, and of course children and young people, to build the evidence of what works, when and for whom.

The youth and wider voluntary and community sector, including organisations led by young people, are a key source of expertise in enabling health professionals to do participation well. Ultimately, participation and engagement that's rich, deep and meaningful, leads to mature models of co-production and it results in lasting change. Whatever our age and situation, society needs us all to become active participants in health and wellbeing; passively receiving care and having services provided cannot be an option. Everyone can contribute; some may need more support than others, but all voices and perspectives, whether at an individual, community, national or global level, have a part to play in mobilising greater participation and engagement in personal health, and in the design and delivery of healthcare. The earlier this participation and engagement process begins the more likely we are to foster that spirit of collaboration and the sense of agency relating to our personal health and wellbeing that is so critical if we are to transform the health and wellbeing of society.

The policy drivers which exist to support this work – the United Nations Convention on the Rights of the Child, NHS Constitution, The Health and Social Care Act, the NHS Long Term plan – all act as our compasses. Our challenge is to bring these to life with the children and young people who are current and future users of health services. This book brings together the evidence base, offers inspiration and encourages us to go further on this journey together. Please dip in and be inspired, but most importantly use the ideas to engage children and young people in your work.

Kath Evans
Children's Nurse and Children's Rights champion

Introduction: embedding young people's participation in healthcare

Louca-Mai Brady

> 'Knowing that I could be part of preventing some of the struggles I had within services, for the next young people coming through them, was what motivated me to get involved in participation. Not only did I want to see changes, but I myself could be part of that change.' Lizzy, young co-author, Chapter 7

The United Nations Convention on the Rights of the Child (UN, 1989: UNCRC) states that all children have a right to the highest possible standards of both healthcare and to have a say in matters that affect them. Involving young people in the commissioning, development and delivery of health services is essential to ensure that these better reflect children and young people's priorities and concerns. There are disparities in who participates, the types of decisions they are involved in making and the extent to which participation is meaningful and effective for both young people and professionals (Davey, 2010; Percy-Smith, 2010). It is also important to consider the forms participation takes and the processes which facilitate that involvement, that is, what young people are involved in and how, and the impact that this has on both services and young people.

This book responds directly to these ideas. In so doing it presents a range of different models and approaches to participation in healthcare practice from the perspectives of people working in the NHS and voluntary sector, researchers and young people. This includes considering young people's participation in shared decision-making (Part I), participation in national projects and programmes (Part II), collaborative research with young people in NHS Trusts (Part III) and young people-led participation (Part IV). These examples present new insights into the realities, challenges and opportunities for young people's participation in healthcare while also providing a critical perspective on current approaches. In the concluding chapter (Chapter 10), a new approach to understanding young people's participation is put forward to inform future thinking and practice.

Young people: a note on terminology

'Childhood' has many and varied definitions including 'the status of being a minor, the early-life state of immaturity whether actual or ascribed and the process of growing towards adulthood' (Alderson, 2013, p 4). In legislation with regard to education and children's services, 'children' are generally understood to be those from birth to 18 (McNeish, 1999) in line with the UNCRC although age ranges vary according to policy domain. For instance, young disabled people, those with special educational needs and some looked after children are often entitled to support until the age of 25. Meanwhile, 'youth' or 'young people' is commonly defined as 13–25 years old in terms of service delivery, but can occasionally include those aged up to 35 (UN, 2016). So, although there is overlap between 'children' and 'young people' the terms are not synonymous. While the participation of all children is important, the focus in this book is on young people of secondary school age (11–18) primarily in the UK healthcare context. However, many of the debates and issues are equally relevant to younger children's participation and this is reflected in reference to both 'children and young people', as well as to 'children's rights' in the context of the UNCRC.

What is 'participation'?

Participation can be at the level of individual decision-making (young people's participation in decisions that affect their own lives, for example with respect to health and care planning) and at a more strategic level (participation in policy and service development). The ways in which we understand participation informs how it is enacted in practice and young people's experiences of being involved (Day et al, 2015; Brady, 2017). The language of participation can be vague and contradictory 'with the same word being used to describe very varied activity in very differing circumstances' (Kirby et al, 2003, p 21). It can be used to mean taking part in an activity, but more commonly is used to refer to involvement in decision-making (Thomas, 2007).

Many models of children's participation make distinctions between levels of participation according to the degree of power that is shared or transferred (Hart, 1992; Shier, 2001). Arnstein's (1971) ladder of citizen participation was adapted by Hart (1992) to include children and young people.

Hart's (1992) ladder is still central to much discussion about young people's participation, with many typologies aiming to either refine Hart's model or set themselves apart

Figure 0.1: Ladder of participation

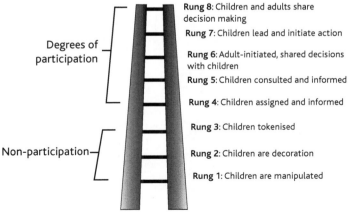

Degrees of participation

Rung 8: Children and adults share decision making

Rung 7: Children lead and initiate action

Rung 6: Adult-initiated, shared decisions with children

Rung 5: Children consulted and informed

Rung 4: Children assigned and informed

Rung 3: Children tokenised

Non-participation

Rung 2: Children are decoration

Rung 1: Children are manipulated

Source: Adapted from Hart (1992, p 8)

from the implication that 'full empowerment' is the ultimate aim of participation (McNeish, 1999; Thomas, 2007). For example, Kirby et al (2003) argue that the type of participation activity should be determined according to circumstances of the participating young people, and that therefore no level of participation is 'better' than another. Likewise, Alderson (2001) proposes that good practice should mean that practitioners ascertain, and continue to check, the level of involvement desired by individual young people rather than assuming any level is inherently better. Indeed, in exploring what 'effective participation' means in healthcare settings, the idea of empowering children as 'experts by experience' in their own lives, needs to be balanced with professional responsibility and expertise. The key point for consideration by readers of this book is that different forms and levels of participation may be appropriate in different circumstances and for different young people.

In this book contributors consider young people's participation in both individual decision-making and at a more strategic level. In addition to understanding participation at the level of individual or strategic decision-making (Kirby et al, 2003), McNeish talks of participation in service development and provision meaning 'the involvement of young people individually or collectively as consumers of services' (1999, p 194). Others distinguish between participation in individual care; participation in communities; participation in services and participation in planning, commissioning and governance (Faulkner et al, 2015). This is echoed by Wright et al (2006) who argue that participation should be based on a circular rather than graduated model of participation, with four key elements:

- children and young people's involvement in individual decisions about their own lives, as well as collective involvement in matters that affect them;
- a culture of listening that enables children and young people to influence decisions about the services they receive as individuals, as well as how those services are developed and delivered;

- not an isolated activity, but an ongoing process by which children and young people are enabled to influence change within an organisation;
- not a hierarchy where the 'aim' is to reach the top…different levels of participation are valid for different groups of children and young people and at different stages of an organisation's development. (Wright et al, 2006, p 9)

While it may indeed be appropriate for the level and nature of participation to be determined by the circumstances of the young people involved, the dominant structures for young people's participation in the NHS generally take the form of collective participation structures such as youth forums and young people's advisory groups (Crowley, 2015). While these can certainly be effective ways for young people to influence decision-making (see Chapter 3), they are often adult-led and may limit opportunities for children and young people to speak out and contribute creatively according to their own agenda, priorities and frames of reference.[1] Cairns (2006) suggests that structures such as youth councils, parliaments, deliberative forums, advisory groups and panels fall within the model of representative democracy (working with small groups of young people as representatives of a wider population) rather than participative democracy (creating opportunities for young people 'to be participants on their own behalf') (p 222). Strategic participation can be individual as well as collective and as such may indeed enable some children and young people to participate who would not otherwise be able to do so (Brady, 2017; Brady et al, 2018b). However, there is a need 'to pay closer attention to who is participating, in what and for whose benefit' (Cornwall, 2008, p 269), and furthermore *how* they are participating. The contributors to this book consider how best to involve young people in meaningful and effective ways, who may be excluded by different approaches, and when alternative approaches may be better.

In their *Handbook of Children and Young People's Participation*, Percy-Smith and Thomas (2010) note that while participation can be understood in terms of influencing decisions and outcomes, evidence from practice across the world illustrates that participation also refers to the *process* by which involvement happens. In this way we can make a distinction between participation and participatory practice – a democratic process in which people work together to find solutions and make decisions (Percy-Smith, 2018) – and is more reflective of the participative research tradition championed by the likes of Reason and Bradbury (2008).

'Participation', 'shared decision-making', 'partnership' and 'inclusion' are often used interchangeably when discussing the involvement of children and young people in health services (McPherson, 2010). 'Patient experience', '(service user) involvement' and 'engagement' are also commonly used terms in many health services, and co-production and co-design are increasingly popular (Batalden et al, 2016; Fugini et al, 2016), although often understood simplistically in terms of *involvement* without reference to issues of power or quality of involvement (Social Care Institute for Excellence (SCIE), 2015).

The starting point for this book is the commonly held understanding of participation as a process by which children and young people influence decisions which bring about change in themselves, their peers, the services they use and their communities (Participation Works, 2010). However, talking about young people 'influencing decisions' does not necessarily denote a transfer of power (Boyden and Ennew, 1997), as it implies only taking part or being present, young people 'having their voices heard' or 'sharing their views', rather than working in collaborative relationships with adults (Percy-Smith, 2016). Kirby (2004) makes the distinction between consultation (seeking the views of young people) and collaboration and user (or youth)-led as more active forms of participation (Sinclair, 2004; Thomas, 2007) in which young people are directly and democratically involved in all stages of the decision-making process (Shier, 2001; Hill et al, 2004).

Why does young people's participation in healthcare matter?

A significant driver for enhancing young people's participation in healthcare and, increasingly, service user involvement is linked to patient experience (McNally et al, 2015). There have also been repeated calls to involve patients and members of the public in healthcare improvement in response to serious clinical and service failings in the UK and internationally (Ocloo and Matthews, 2016). As a result, children and young people's participation is an increasing priority in many healthcare organisations (Weil et al, 2015). Involving children and young people in the commissioning, development and delivery of health services should ensure that these better reflect children and young people's needs and concerns as well as improving their care experience. Global evidence for children and young people's participation in health services is growing rapidly, and international examples of good practice include the Youth Friendly Hospital Programme in Australia, Give Youth a Voice in Canada (Weil et al, 2015), the World Health Organization's *Adolescent friendly health services: An agenda for change* (WHO, 2002) and the *Council of Europe guidelines on child-friendly healthcare* (CoE Committee of Ministers, 2011). There is an expectation inherent in the UK NHS Constitution 'that patients, service users and the public participate nationally and locally in the development, implementation and accountability processes of health and social care policy and services' (Davies, 2013, p 2). The Chief Medical Officer's 2013 report emphasised the importance of the UNCRC to these participation processes and said that:

> This expectation for patient and public participation has no age limit. Children and young people … should be encouraged and facilitated to participate in decisions about their own care and, more broadly, about the health and social care services and policies that affect them. (Davies, 2013, p 2)

English legislation and policy have to some extent reflected these expectations: in the health sector participation has been given momentum as a result of legislation including the Children Act (2004), Children and Families Act (2014) and the Health and Social Care Act (2012), policy reports including the *Kennedy Report* (Kennedy, 2010); the *National service framework: children, young people and maternity services* (DHSC, 2004); *Our health, our care, our say* (DHSC, 2006) and the *NHS Long Term Plan* (NHS England, 2019). Alongside this there has been increasing awareness of the importance of developing children and young people's participation in health services in a strategic and systematic way (Association for Young People's Health (AYPH), 2010; Davies, 2013). There has also been increased use of rights-based tools and quality criteria such as *Hear by Right* (Badham and Wade, 2008) and the *You're welcome – Quality criteria for young people friendly health services* (DHSC, 2011; being updated at the time of writing). Other national developments in England have included NHS England establishing a Youth Forum (see Chapter 3), the work of the Royal College of Paediatrics and Child Health 'RCPCH &Us' network (Chapter 4), the introduction of new children's experience measures within the NHS (Hargreaves et al, 2019), the Care Quality Commission involving children in their inspection activities,[2] and the involvement of children on the board of Healthwatch England and within local Healthwatch bodies (DHSC, 2013). There is evidence that health services that are co-produced with children and young people are more likely to be well utilised, result in better patient experience, better outcomes and provide better value for money (Heimer et al, 2018; Reddy, 2018). Young people's participation in healthcare therefore also makes economic sense. Accordingly, organisations like the Association for Young People's Health (Chapter 5), Investing in Children (Chapter 8), Common Room (Chapter 1)[3] and Redthread[4] are developing exciting projects in collaboration with, or led by young people.

A further influence on participation in healthcare is that all publicly funded health research in the UK is now expected to have some element of public involvement (Evans et al, 2014). Involving those who are the focus of health research has been found to have a positive impact on what is researched and the impact of research findings on services and in the lives of those involved (Staley, 2009; Brett et al, 2014). Research which actively involves young people, if used to inform healthcare decision-making or policy formulation, should lead to policies and services that better reflect children and young people's priorities and concerns (Fleming and Boeck, 2012; Brady et al, 2018a) and enhance the opportunity for optimal health outcomes (Jamal et al, 2014).

The gap between rhetoric and reality

In spite of the rationale outlined earlier, in reality paediatric services are seen as the 'poor relation' to adult services within the NHS (Evans, 2016), and children and young people are largely invisible within most NHS all-age programmes (Viner, 2018). The result is that NHS care typically results in worse patient experience and lower quality care for children and young people than for adults (Hargreaves et al, 2019). Children and young people in the UK suffer worse health and wellbeing outcomes than their peers in comparable countries across a range of physical and mental health measures, including overall mortality and deaths from long-term conditions such as epilepsy, asthma and diabetes (Davies, 2013; Viner et al, 2017). A recent Children's Rights Alliance for England briefing on the state of children's rights in health (CRAE, 2018a) highlighted the need for improvements in child and adolescent mental health support and concerns about the impact of inequalities and Brexit on children and young people's health. In order to better meet children and young people's needs health services need to be developed and delivered in a child-friendly way and with an understanding of their needs (Care Quality Commission (CQC), 2018; Royal College of Paediatrics and Child Health (RCPCH), 2019). However, as Kath Evans highlights in the Foreword to this book, young people's participation goes beyond improving healthcare; it is also important in terms of young people's sense of agency and actorship as citizens and members of communities including health communities.

There is a lack of evidence about how the apparent commitment to participation and children's rights translates into professional practice and young people's experience of participation in health services (Day et al, 2015). There is also a lack of evidence on whether and how children's rights are enabled in local practice, and whether this has necessarily led to improved outcomes for children (Ferguson, 2013), or on policymaking and service delivery (Byrne and Lundy, 2015; Crowley, 2015). A recent assessment of the state of children's rights in England found that children and young people are still not systematically involved in national decision-making, and the extent to which children and young people are listened to by professionals often relies on the commitment of individuals (CRAE, 2018b). Despite children and young people's participation having an increasingly high profile in healthcare, in practice it is limited and patchy (RCPCH, 2010; Blades et al, 2013). Young people's participation faces many challenges in the face of the realities of clinical practice: the values and ideologies of professionals, organisational systems and processes can be at odds with the priorities and concerns of children and young people, but with adult professionals having the power to enable or potentially constrain children and young people's participation (Brady, 2017). Children and young people are 'generally excluded and not sufficiently involved in individual healthcare decisions, [...] service improvement and policy-making' (Ehrich, et al, 2015, p 783). This can mean a focus on consultation with children about their individual health needs rather than participation in the commissioning, delivery or evaluation of health services, or in the development of health policy (Blades et al, 2013; Brady et al, 2018a).

Structures and processes of participation

The case for young people's participation is well established (for example Kirby et al, 2003; Percy-Smith and Thomas, 2010), but it is a multi-layered (Sinclair, 2004) and sometimes contested concept (Lansdown, 2006) with multiple interpretations in practice. A wide range of models, toolkits and 'how to' guides have been influential both in promoting children and young people's participation and documenting where it is lacking (Kirby, 2004; Tisdall et al, 2014). But the theory and models underpinning the practice of participation often appear confused and contradictory (Thomas, 2007; Malone and Hartung, 2010). There is a need to consider how and when young people participate, accommodating 'new kinds of participatory practice' and understanding institutional context and processes 'and the cultures and dispositions that underpin them' (Thomas, 2007, pp 215–16). However, the predominant focus hitherto on hearing children's views has placed the emphasis on the input of individual children and young people without explicitly acknowledging the role of organisational cultures and processes in enabling change to happen (Kirby et al, 2003; Wright et al, 2006; Tisdall et al, 2014; Brady, 2017) or the importance of integrating children's participation into service evaluation and improvement (Percy-Smith, 2010). A key focus for this book therefore is how understandings of participation, cultures, processes and practice enable or create barriers to young people's participation being embedded in healthcare practice and policy.

Rights and responsibilities

Children's rights both in relation to decisions about their own healthcare and concerning the development of services are underpinned by the UNCRC ratified by the UK government in 1991. The UNCRC encompasses social, economic, civil and political rights, and 'asserts children's right to have a voice in decision-making, as well as rights to freedom of thought and expression' (Percy-Smith and Thomas, 2010, p 1). The key article relating to participation, Article 12, states that:

> States Parties shall assure to the child who is capable of forming his or her own views the right to express those views freely in all matters affecting the child, the views of the child being given due weight in accordance with the age and maturity of the child. (UN, 1989)

Children's rights apply to children and young people as individuals and as a constituency (that is, representing other children and young people, for example in an advisory group). A key implication of Article 24 of the UNCRC is that all children and young people have needs that must be met in order to optimise their health and wellbeing:

> States Parties recognize the right of the child to the enjoyment of the highest attainable standard of

health and to facilities for the treatment of illness and rehabilitation of health. States Parties shall strive to ensure that no child is deprived of his or her right of access to such health care services. (UN, 1989)

In a General Comment on Article 24, which sets out how that article should be interpreted by signatories to the UNCRC, the UN Committee on the Rights of the Child emphasises 'the importance of approaching children's health from a child-rights perspective' (UN, 2013, p 3) and states that:

> Article 12 highlights the importance of children's participation …. This includes their views on all aspects of health provisions, including, for example, what services are needed, how and where they are best provided, barriers to accessing or using services, the quality of the services and the attitudes of health professionals, how to strengthen children's capacities to take increasing levels of responsibility for their own health and development, and how to involve them more effectively in the provision of services, as peer educators. States are encouraged to conduct regular participatory consultations, which are adapted to the age and maturity of the child, and research with children, and to do this separately with their parents, in order to learn about their health challenges, developmental needs and expectations as a contribution to the design of effective interventions and health programmes. (UN, 2013, p 7)

This quotation sets out in far more detail than the UNCRC itself what children's rights under Article 24 mean for young people's participation in health services both within decisions about their own care and in collaborative and strategic participation. It also highlights what the UN Committee thinks successful participation in health services and research might look like in practice. The realisation of children's rights to health, and to participation, requires their translation into policy and practice; as well as children and young people's participation in conceptualising and realising these rights (Spronk, 2014). In doing so this rights-based rationale for young people's participation in health policy and practice makes a direct link between children's involvement and patient benefit.

Participation rights do not operate in a vacuum, and the UN General Comment on Article 24 quoted earlier emphasises the interdependency of children's rights. The UNCRC recognises that children and young people 'also have particular needs and vulnerabilities that require special protection beyond the rights to which adults are entitled' (Groundwater-Smith et al, 2015, p 6), and sets out the responsibilities of adults to provide guidance to children and young people and to protect them from harm (McNeish, 1999). Tensions inherent in the UNCRC between participation, protection and provision rights can be particularly acute in relation to children and young people's health (Franklin and Sloper, 2005; Alderson, 2014) and between children's rights and wellbeing (Tisdall, 2015), for example when healthcare practitioners have to strike a balance between children and young people's rights and clinical responsibilities (Schalkers et al, 2016). Tensions between provision and protection rights and participation rights can be particularly acute in relation to children and young people's participation in decisions about their individual care as healthcare organisations are:

> often steeped in welfare principles which view children as essentially vulnerable and lacking competence and adults as responsible for their care and protection. (McNeish, 1999, p 193)

In health services, adults often 'take a protective stance towards children to act in their best interest' (Coyne and Harder, 2011, p 312). Such stances may be based on ideas about children and young people's competence or adults taking the view that children and young people's participation in decision-making processes is potentially disruptive to their wellbeing (Vis et al, 2011). But health professionals, and parents and carers, do have duties to protect and provide developmental opportunities for the children and young people for whom they are responsible. The challenge for young people's participation is when adults impose their own perspectives, consciously or unconsciously, on young people or have different perspectives on what is in a young person's best interests (Ehrich et al, 2015). If young people's views are seen as less important, or less valid, than adults' views this will influence practices and approaches towards them, with the result that young people's participation at best becomes tokenistic and at worst, becomes a lost opportunity for informing how health services can respect the views and insights of young people as citizens and effectively respond to their needs.

But protection and provision rights can enhance, as well as challenge, participation rights:

> The health service has a child's survival and development rights as its key focus, but all those working with children within a service need to ensure children's rights to protection and participation are also given equal consideration ... in the context of children being part of a wider society that also has needs and rights. (Jones and Welch, 2010, p 167)

This consideration of competing for complementary rights and the implications for children and young people's participation in health services is picked up by several of the chapters which follow.

Who participates?

'Young people' are not a homogenous group. Apart from age, this 'group' varies immensely by ethnicity, culture, disability, gender, socio-economic situation, living circumstances and many other factors, with associated variation in access to services and opportunities. There are disparities in the characteristics of young people likely to participate, the types of decisions they are involved in making, and the extent to which this participation is meaningful and effective (Cockburn, 2005; Percy-Smith, 2010). The mechanisms of formal participation may also privilege the already privileged (Crowley, 2015). This is reflected in uncertainty about 'how to involve a diversity of patients and the public, rather than a few selected individuals' in healthcare (Ocloo and Matthews, 2016, p 2). Disabled young people and looked after children, among other 'less frequently heard' groups, are still not routinely or systematically involved in individual or strategic decision-making in health services (CRAE, 2015a; CRAE, 2015b; Alderson et al, 2019). Indeed, those with greater healthcare needs are also often those 'most excluded from healthcare decision-making' (Ocloo and Matthews, 2016, p 4) and frequently less likely to be involved in decisions about their own care. Young people who, due to a combination of their circumstances and lived experiences come to be identified as 'vulnerable' or 'disadvantaged,' are likely to experience more barriers to participation while conversely being those that health organisations may be failing to reach (McNeish, 1999). It is important to consider both how to increase the diversity of young people's participation in health services and when it might be more appropriate to involve 'a few selected individuals', for example those with particular lived experience relevant to a service or project. Youth forums and advisory groups can be an effective way to involve young people and offer them a chance to gain skills and experience as well as a chance to contribute to a range of projects and programmes. But they don't work for all young people or all services and projects and can unintentionally marginalise some (Brady, 2017; Brady et al, 2018b). Hence structures of participation can privilege the voices of the few while marginalising the participation of the majority.

Power and control

Young people's participation in health services takes place within the context of epistemological shifts in the role of the medical specialist and the development of models of shared decision-making (Ocloo and Matthews, 2016). But there is an additional power dimension in that young people's participation in the UK still tends to focus on adult-initiated participation within a formal setting. In order to participate fully, young people need to be respected as rights-holders, but also for there to be 'mutual esteem and solidarity, and a sense of shared purpose'

(Thomas, 2012, p 463). However, there are 'inequalities and injustices in the way power is exercised and decision-making controlled by adults' (Percy-Smith, 2016, p 401; UN, 2013). While inviting children to contribute in adult-initiated agenda might be useful and have impact in development of national and local NHS services, this is quite a different ethos to participatory learning and change characterised by a more democratic process involving collaboration, dialogue and co-inquiry/co-production to challenge and change systems and practices (Percy-Smith, 2016). This book explores ideas of young people as change agents and active citizens, and how this could inform more collaborative and young person-centred participatory practice (Malone and Hartung, 2010; Nolas, 2015).

The focus and structure of this book

This book grew out of participatory research which identified the need for a critical perspective on current approaches to young people's participation in healthcare settings and examples of more participatory and inclusive practice (Brady, 2017). The book explores:

- initiatives where projects have sought to grapple with and respond to the issues set out in this Introduction and in doing so provide examples of good participatory practice with young people;
- how stated commitments to participation and 'child voice' can best translate into changes in systems, practices and young people's experience of participation and of health services;
- how healthcare cultures, systems and processes can support or create barriers to the embedding of young people's participation;
- ways in which participation in health services can transfer more power to young people, and also include more of the young people most likely to use health services;
- the potential for young people-led approaches to participation in healthcare.

Structure

Part I considers young people's participation in individual decision-making. Chapter 1 explores the potential, and challenges, for shared decision-making with young people about their mental healthcare. Chapter 2 discusses the participation of disabled young people in end-of-life healthcare decisions. The latter powerfully highlights why young people's participation is not just a nice thing to do, or a legal obligation, but can be a matter of life and death.

Part II considers young people's participation in national projects and programmes. Chapter 3 discusses the background and development of youth forums and councils in the NHS, and reflects on lessons from an evaluation of the NHS England Youth Forum. Chapter 4 explores how the 'RCPCH & Us' network and Engagement Collaborative supports children, young people and families to influence and shape health policy and practice. In Chapter 5 the Association for Young People's Health discuss the innovative ways in which they have engaged young people whose voices are less heard in the development of youth-friendly health services.

Part III discusses the learning from two collaborative action research projects in NHS services. Chapter 6 shares the experience of developing meaningful and effective opportunities for involving children and young people across an NHS Trust, critically reflecting on the significance of participation as patient experience and the challenges of integrating children's participation into organisational culture and systems. Chapter 7 discusses learning from a project which sought to develop and embed participation across a group of children's community health services. It also considers the implications of the organisation's subsequent recommissioning for young people's participation, illustrating how participation is in turn affected by wider systems change.

Part IV explores two examples of young people-led participation. Chapter 8 explores the work of Investing in Children, highlighting in particular the benefits and challenges of working collaboratively to enable young people to become agents in the creation of new ways of working. Chapter 9 discusses the work of RAiISE: a young person–led charity which aims to improve care for young people living with invisible illnesses, a great example of young people leading a health and wellbeing initiative with the support of healthcare and education professionals.

In the concluding chapter (Chapter 10) the editor draws on the learning from the preceding chapters and her own research, to present a new rights-based framework for embedding children and young people's participation in practice.

Postscript

During the period in which this book was being edited the NHS, and indeed the whole world, was upended by the COVID-19 pandemic. The longer-term implications of this for health services and young people's participation are as yet unknown, but there are short-term implications in the context of this book. Some participation has continued, albeit mainly online, which has implications for who is able to be involved. For some young people online involvement can be more accessible than travelling to meetings and events, but digital exclusion and the accessibility of many online platforms can also exclude others. This presents challenges but also opportunities to develop and learn from new ways of involving young people. But at the same time participation and public involvement have often had to 'take a back seat' while health services have been dealing with an unprecedented crisis. While this is understandable, there is a risk that, far from being embedded, participation could fall back into being a 'nice thing to do if you have time'. We need to guard against that and, as Kath said in the Foreword, continue on this journey together. It is more important now than ever that young people's participation is embedded into the design and delivery of health services. The challenges of COVID-19 have highlighted the potential to do things differently, and develop more participatory and inclusive practice in collaboration with young people.

Notes

[1]   See Percy-Smith (2007) for ways that young people can participate in more creative and empowering ways.

[2]   www.cqc.org.uk/content/how-we-involve-you
[3]   http://commonroom.uk.com/
[4]   www.redthread.org.uk/

References

Alderson, H., Brown, R., Smart, D., Lingam, R. and Dovey-Pearce, G. (2019) 'You've come to children that are in care and given us the opportunity to get our voices heard': The journey of looked after children and researchers in developing a Patient and Public Involvement group. *Health Expectations*, 22 (4), pp 657–65.

Alderson, P. (2001) Research by children. *International Journal of Social Research Methodology*, 4 (2), pp 139–53.

Alderson, P. (2013) *Childhoods Real and Imagined. Volume 1: An Introduction to Critical Realism and Childhood Studies*. London: Routledge.

Alderson, P. (2014) Children as patients. In G.B. Melton, A. Ben-Arieh, J. Cashmore, G.S. Goodman and N.K. Worley (eds.) *The Sage Handbook of Child Research*. London: SAGE, pp 100–17.

Arnstein, S. (1971) A ladder of citizen participation. *Journal of the American Institute of Planners*, 35 (4) pp 216–24.

Association for Young People's Health (AYPH) (2010) *Involving young people in the development of health services*. London: Association for Young People's Health. Available from: www.ayph.org.uk/publications/50_BriefingPaperI.pdf

Badham, B. and Wade, H. (2008) *Hear by Right: Standards Framework for the Participation of Children and Young People*. Revised edition. Leicester: National Youth Agency.

Batalden, M., Batalden, P. and Margolis, P. (2016) Coproduction of healthcare service. *BMJ Quality and Safety*, 25 (7) pp 509–17.

Blades, R., Renton, Z., La Valle, I., Clements, K., Gibb, J. and Lea, J. (2013) '*We would like to make a change': Children and young people's participation in strategic health decision-making*. London: Office of the Children's Commissioner. Available from: www.childrenscommissioner.gov.uk/publication/we-would-like-to-make-a-change/

Boyden, J. and Ennew, J. (1997) *Children in Focus: A Manual for Participatory Research with Children*. Stockholm: Radda Barnen.

Brady, L.M. (2017) *Rhetoric to reality: An inquiry into embedding young people's participation in health services and research*. PhD, University of the West of England. Available from: http://eprints.uwe.ac.uk/29885

Brady, L.M., Hathway, F. and Roberts, R. (2018a) A case study of children's participation in health policy and practice. In P. Beresford and S. Carr (eds.) (2018) *Social Policy First Hand*. Bristol: Policy Press, pp 62–73.

Brady, L.M., Templeton, L., Toner, P., Watson, J., Evans, D., Percy-Smith, B. and Copello, A. (2018b) Involving young people in drug and alcohol research. *Drugs and Alcohol Today*, 18 (1), pp 28–38.

Brett, J., Staniszewska, S., Mockford, C., Herron-Marx, S., Hughes, J., Tysall, C. and Suleman, R. (2014) Mapping the impact of patient and public involvement on health and social care research: A systematic review. *Health Expectations*, 17 (5), pp 637–50.

Byrne, B. and Lundy, L. (2015) Reconciling children's policy and children's rights: Barriers to effective government delivery. *Children & Society*, 29 (4), pp 266–76.

Cairns, L. (2006) Participation with purpose – The right to be heard. In E.K.M. Tisdall, J.M. Davis, M. Hill and A. Prout (eds.) *Children, Young People and Social Inclusion: Participation for What?* Bristol: Policy Press, pp 217–34.

Care Quality Commission (CQC) (2018) *2018 Children and young people's inpatient and day case survey*. Available from: www.cqc.org.uk/publications/surveys/children-young-peoples-survey-2016

CRAE (Children's Rights Alliance for England) (2015a) *UK implementation of the UN Convention on the rights of the child: Civil society alternative report 2015 to the UN Committee – England*. London: CRAE. Available from: www.crae.org.uk/news/crae-submits-two-child-rights-reports-to-un/

CRAE (2015b) *See it, say it, change it: Submission to the UN Committee on the rights of the child*. London: CRAE. Available from: http://www.crae.org.uk/media/119341/crae_seeit-sayit-changeit_web.pdf

CRAE (2018a) *State of children's rights in England. 7: Health.* London: CRAE. Available from: www.crae.org.uk/media/126997/B7_CRAE_HEALTH_WEB.pdf

CRAE (2018b) *State of children's rights in England.* London: CRAE. Available from: www.crae.org.uk/our-work/monitoring-compliance-with-childrens-rights/state-of-childrens-rights-in-england/

Cockburn, T. (2005) Children's participation in social policy: Inclusion, chimera or authenticity? *Social Policy and Society*, 4 (2), pp 109–19.

Cornwall, A. (2008) Unpacking 'participation': Models, meanings and practices. *Community Development Journal*, 43 (3), pp 269–83.

Council of Europe (CoE) Committee of Ministers (2011) *Council of Europe guidelines on child-friendly health care.* Available from: www.coe.int/en/web/children/child-friendly-healthcare

Coyne, I. and Harder, M. (2011) Children's participation in decision-making: Balancing protection with shared decision-making using a situational perspective. *Journal of Child Health Care*, 15 (4), pp 312–19.

Crowley, A. (2015) Is anyone listening? The impact of children's participation on public policy. *International Journal of Children's Rights*, 23 (3), pp 602–21.

Davey, C. (2010) *Children's participation in decision-making: A summary report on progress made up to 2010.* London: National Children's Bureau.

Davies, S. (2013) *Chief Medical Officer's annual report 2012: Our children deserve better: Prevention pays.* Available from: www.gov.uk/government/publications/chief-medical-officers-annual-report-2012-our-children-deserve-better-prevention-pays

Day, L., Percy-Smith, B., Ruxton, R., McKenna, K., Redgrave, K. and Young, T. (2015) *Evaluation of legislation, policy and practice of child participation in the European Union (EU).* Brussels: DG Justice Available from: http://bookshop.europa.eu/en/evaluation-of-legislation-policy-and-practice-of-child-participation-in-the-european-union-eu--pbDS0514101/?CatalogCategoryID=cOwKABstC3oAAAEjeJEY4e5L

Department of Health and Social Care (2004) *National service framework: Children, young people and maternity services*. Available from: www.gov.uk/government/publications/national-service-framework-children-young-people-and-maternity-services

Department of Health and Social Care (2006) *Our health, our care, our say: A new direction for community services*. Available from: www.gov.uk/government/publications/our-health-our-care-our-say-a-new-direction-for-community-services

Department of Health and Social Care (2011) *You're welcome – Quality criteria for young people friendly health services*. Available from: www.gov.uk/government/publications/quality-criteria-for-young-people-friendly-health-services

Department of Health and Social Care (2013) *Improving children and young people's health outcomes: A system wide response*. Available from: www.gov.uk/government/uploads/system/uploads/attachment_data/file/214928/9328-TSO-2900598-DH-SystemWideResponse.pdf

Ehrich, J., Pettoello-Mantovani, M., Lenton, S., Damm, L. and Goldhagen, J. (2015) Participation of children and young people in their health care: Understanding the potential and limitations. *Journal of Pediatrics*, 167 (3), pp 783–4.

Evans, D., Coad, J., Cottrell, K., Dalrymple, J., Davies, R., Donald, C., Laterza, V., Long, A., Longley, A., Moule, P., Pollard, K., Powell, J., Puddicombe, A.R., Rice, C. and Sayers, R. (2014) Public involvement in research: Assessing impact through a realist evaluation. *Health Services and Delivery Research*, 2 (36), pp 1–128.

Evans, K. (2016) Listen and learn. *Journal of Family Health*, 26 (3), pp 44–6.

Faulkner, A., Yiannoullou, S., Kalathil, J., Crepaz-Keay, D., Singer, F., James, N., Griffiths, R., Perry, E., Forde, D. and Kallevik, J. (2015) *Involvement for influence: 4Pi National Involvement Standards*. London: National Survivor User Network (NSUN) [online]. Available from: https://www.nsun.org.uk/faqs/4pi-national-involvement-standards

Ferguson, L. (2013) Not merely rights for children but children's rights: The theory gap and the assumption of the importance of children's rights. *The International Journal of Children's Rights*, 21 (2), pp 177–208.

Fleming, J. and Boeck, T. (eds.) (2012) *Involving Children and Young People in Health and Social Care Research*. London: Routledge.

Franklin, A. and Sloper, P. (2005) Listening and responding? Children's participation in health care within England. *International Journal of Children's Rights*. 13, pp 11–29.

Fugini, M., Bracci, E. and Sicilia, M. (eds.) (2016) *Co-production in the Public Sector: Experiences and Challenges*. London: Springer.

Groundwater-Smith, S., Dockett, S. and Bottrell, D. (2015) *Participatory Research with Children and Young People*. London: SAGE.

Hargreaves, D.S., Lemer, C., Ewing, C., Cornish, J., Baker, T., Toma, K., Saxena, S., McCulloch, B., McFarlane, L., Welch, J., Sparrow, E., Kossarova, L., Lumsden, D.E., Ronny, C. and Cheung, L.H. (2019) Measuring and improving the quality of NHS care for children and young people. *Archives of Disease in Childhood*, 104 (7), pp 618–21.

Hart, R. A. (1992) *Children's Participation: From Tokenism to Citizenship*. Innocenti Essays 4. Florence: UNICEF International Child Development Centre.

Heimer, M., Näsman, E. and Palme, J. (2018) Vulnerable children's rights to participation, protection, and provision: The process of defining the problem in Swedish child and family welfare. *Child & Family Social Work*, 23 (2), 316–23.

Hill, M., Davis, J., Prout, A. and Tisdall, K. (2004) Moving the participation agenda forward. *Children & Society*, 18 (2), pp 77–96.

Jamal, F., Langford, R., Daniels, P., Thomas, J., Harden, A. and Bonell, C. (2014) Consulting with young people to inform systematic reviews: An example from a review on the effects of schools on health. *Health Expectations*, 18 (6), pp 3225–35.

Jones, P. and Welch, S. (2010) *Rethinking Children's Rights: Attitudes in Contemporary Society*. London: Bloomsbury.

Kennedy, I. (2010) *Getting it right for children and young people: Overcoming cultural barriers in the NHS so as to meet their needs*. London: DHSC. Available from: https://www.gov.uk/government/publications/getting-it-right-for-children-and-young-people-overcoming-cultural-barriers-in-the-nhs-so-as-to-meet-their-needs

Kirby, P. (2004) *A guide to actively involving young people in research: For researchers, research commissioners and managers.* Southampton: INVOLVE. Available from: https://www.invo.org.uk/posttypepublication/a-guide-to-actively-involving-young-people-in-research/

Kirby, P., Lanyon, C., Cronin, K. and Sinclair, R. (2003) *Building a culture of participation: Involving children and young people in policy, service planning, delivery and evaluation.* (Report and Handbook) London: DfES.

Lansdown, G. (2006) International developments in children's participation: lessons and challenges. In K. Tisdall, J. Davis, M. Hill and A. Prout (eds.) (2006) *Children, Young People and Social Inclusion: Participation For What?.* Bristol: Policy Press, pp 139–58.

Malone, K. and Hartung, C. (2010) Challenges of participatory practice with children. In B. Percy-Smith and N. Thomas (eds.) (2010) *A Handbook of Children and Young People's Participation: Perspectives from Theory and Practice.* London: Routledge, pp 24–38.

McNally, D., Sharples, S. and Craig, G. (2015) Patient leadership: Taking patient experience to the next level? *Patient Experience Journal,* 2 (2), pp 7–15.

McNeish, D. (1999) Promoting participation for children and young people: Some key questions for health and social welfare organisations. *Journal of Social Work Practice,* 13 (2), pp 191–204.

McPherson, A. (2010) Involving children: Why it matters. In S. Redsell and A. Hastings (eds.) (2010) *Listening to Children and Young People in Healthcare Consultations.* Oxford: Radcliffe Publishing, pp 15–29.

NHS England (2019) *The NHS Long Term Plan.* London: NHS England. Available from: www.longtermplan.nhs.uk/publication/nhs-long-term-plan/

Nolas, S.-M. (2015) Children's participation, childhood publics and social change: A review. *Children & Society,* 29 (2), pp 157–67.

Ocloo, J. and Matthews, R. (2016) From tokenism to empowerment: Progressing patient and public involvement in healthcare improvement. *BMJ Quality and Safety* 25 (8), pp 1–7. Available from: http://qualitysafety.bmj.com/content/early/2016/03/18/bmjqs-2015–004839.abstract

Participation Works (2010) *Listen and Change: A guide to children and young people's participation rights.* 2nd edition. London: Participation Works. Available from: www.crae.org.uk/publications-resources/listen-and-change-a-guide-to-children-and-young-peoples-participation-rights-(2nd-ed)/

Percy-Smith, B. (2007) "You think you know? ... You have no idea": youth participation in health policy development. *Health Education Research*, 22 (6), pp 879–94.

Percy-Smith, B. (2010) Councils, consultation and community: Rethinking the spaces for children and young people's participation. *Children's Geographies*, 8 (2), pp 107–22.

Percy-Smith, B. (2016) Negotiating active citizenship: Young people's participation in everyday spaces. In K.P. Kallio, S. Mills and T. Skelton (eds.) (2016) *Politics, Citizenship and Rights.* Singapore: Springer Singapore, pp 401–22.

Percy-Smith, B. (2018) Participation as learning for change in everyday spaces: Enhancing meaning and effectiveness using action research. In Baraldi, C. and Cockburn, T. (eds.) *Theorising Childhood: Citizenship, Rights and Participation.* London: Palgrave Macmillan.

Percy-Smith, B. and Thomas, N. (eds.) (2010) *A Handbook of Children's Participation: Perspectives from Theory and Practice.* London: Routledge.

RCPCH (2010) *Not just a phase: A guide to the participation of children and young people in health services.* London: Royal College of Paediatrics and Child Health. Available from: www.rcpch.ac.uk/resources/not-just-phase-guide-participation-children-young-people-health-services

RCPCH (2019) *Rights matter – What the UN Convention on the Rights of the Child means to us.* London: Royal College of Paediatrics and Child Health. Available from: www.rcpch.ac.uk/resources/rights-matter-what-un-convention-rights-child-means-us

Reason, P. and Bradbury, H. (2008) Introduction. In Reason, P. and Bradbury, H. (eds.) *The SAGE Handbook of Action Research: Participative Inquiry and Practice*. 2nd ed. London: SAGE, pp 1–10.

Reddy, V. (2018) Involving families in service redesign. *Paediatrics and Child Health*, 28 (2), pp 100–2.

Schalkers, I., Parsons, C.S., Bunders, J.F. and Dedding, C. (2016) Health professionals' perspectives on children's and young people's participation in health care: A qualitative multihospital study. *Journal of Clinical Nursing*, 25 (7–8), pp 1035–44.

Shier, H. (2001) Pathways to participation: Openings, opportunities and obligations. *Children & Society*. 15 (2), pp 107–17.

Sinclair, R. (2004) Participation in practice: Making it meaningful, effective and sustainable. *Children & Society*. 18 (2), pp 106–18.

Social Care Institute for Excellence (SCIE) (2015) *Co-production in social care: What it is and how to do it*. Available from: https://www.scie.org.uk/publications/guides/guide51/

Spronk, S. (2014) Realizing children's right to health. *International Journal of Children's Rights*, 22 (1), pp 189–204.

Staley, K. (2009) *Exploring impact: Public involvement in NHS, public health and social care research*. Southampton: INVOLVE. Available from: www.invo.org.uk/posttypepublication/exploring-impact-public-involvement-in-nhs-public-health-and-social-care-research/

Thomas, N. (2007) Towards a theory of children's participation. *The International Journal of Children's Rights*, 15 (2), pp 199–218.

Thomas, N. (2012) Love, rights and solidarity: Studying children's participation using Honneth's theory of recognition. *Childhood*, 19 (4), pp 453–66.

Tisdall, E.K.M. (2015) Children's wellbeing and children's rights in tension? *International Journal of Children's Rights*, 23 (4), pp 769–89.

Tisdall, E.K.M., Hinton, R., Gadda, A.M. and Butler, U.M. (2014) Introduction: Children and young people's participation in collective decision-making. In E.K.M. Tisdall, A.M. Gadda and U.M. Butler (eds.) (2014) *Children and Young People's Participation and Its Transformative Potential: Learning from across Countries*. London: Palgrave Macmillan, pp 1–21.

UN (United Nations) (1989) *Convention on the Rights of the Child.* Available from: www.ohchr.org/EN/ProfessionalInterest/ Pages/CRC.aspx

UN (2013) Committee on the Rights of the Child. General Comment No. 15 (2013) on the right of the child to the enjoyment of the highest attainable standard of health (art. 24). Available from: http://tbinternet.ohchr.org/_layouts/ treatybodyexternal/TBSearch.aspx?Lang=enandTreatyID=5 andDocTypeID=11

UN (2016) *Definition of youth.* Available from: https://www. un.org/esa/socdev/documents/youth/fact-sheets/youth- definition.pdf

Viner, R.M., Ashe, M., Cummins, L., Donnellan, M., Friedemann Smith, C., Kitsell, J., Lok, W., Oyinlola, J., Pall, K., Rossiter, A., Stiller, C., de Sa, J. and Pritchard-Jones, K. (2017) *State of child health: Report 2017.* Royal College of Paediatrics and Child Health. Available from: www.rcpch.ac.uk/resources/ state-child-health-2017-full-report

Viner, R.M. (2018) NHS must prioritise health of children and young people. *BMJ* 360. Available from: https://doi. org/10.1136/bmj.k1116

Vis, S.A., Strandbu, A., Holtan, A. and Thomas, N. (2011) Participation and health – a research review of child participation in planning and decision-making. *Child and Family Social Work*, 16 (3), pp 325–35.

Weil, L.G., Lemer, C., Webb, E. and Hargreaves, D.S. (2015) The voices of children and young people in health: Where are we now? *Archives of Disease in Childhood.* 100 (10), pp 915–19.

WHO (2002) *Adolescent friendly health services: An agenda for change.* Geneva: World Health Organization. Available from: www.who.int/maternal_child_adolescent/documents/fch_ cah_02_14/en/

Wright, P., Turner, C., Clay, D. and Mills, H. (2006) *Involving children and young people in developing social care.* Participation Practice Guide 06, London: SCIE. Available from: www.scie. org.uk/publications/guides/guide11/

PART I

Young people's participation in individual decision-making

1

Shared decision-making with young people in mental health services

Kate Martin and Amy Feltham

This chapter explores shared decision-making with young people about their mental healthcare. This includes:

- a foreword from a young adult with experience of using inpatient services about the meaning of shared decision-making;
- the constraints on shared decision-making in mental health inpatient units;
- tools and resources to support shared decision-making.

Foreword from Amy

I am not normally as candid about my personal experience as I have been in this chapter. In general, I use professional experience and the views of the young people of today. However, when I read the first draft, I found that the experiences young people of today mirror my memories of inpatient units. As I have the benefit of hindsight, it felt important to give my own experiences as a patient as part of my contribution to this chapter.

I was 16 when I first came across shared decision-making. I'd dropped out of school and work and was in and out of Child and Adolescent Mental Health (CAMHS) inpatient services like a yo-yo. Through voluntary work, I had found myself on the steering group for a Health Foundation-funded project called 'Closing the Gap: Shared Decision Making in CAMHS'.[1] I was sat in a room full of very highly skilled professionals, advocates and research fellows and yet I was lost. I couldn't understand what shared decision-making was, or what I was doing there. Despite their best efforts, no one in the room could explain the concept. I'd been battered about in the mental health system for years. Shared decision-making wasn't something I'd come across. To my mind, the professionals were the experts and they decided what happened. My doctors negotiated with my parents and I was presented with the results of this decision-making process. This made perfect sense, the doctors held the prescription pads and keys to the ward, and my parents were in charge of what I could and couldn't do at home. What on earth did 'Shared Decision-Making' mean? Why would anyone involve me?

The less choice I felt I had, the more I crumbled into impulsivity, with no visible modelling of rational decision-making. I felt less and less identity, more like a pawn in some tactical game of chess. Everyone wanted me to win, to get to the other side of the chessboard, but I wasn't involved in how this happened. I awaited my recovery, thinking it must be my rebellions against my parents and professionals that meant I was not reaching it. But the more I attended the steering groups the more I understood shared decision-making. It was a whole new world, and one that I increasingly saw the need for.

Ten years later, shared decision-making has shaped my life more than I ever expected. I work as a project engagement worker for an independent organisation that supports shared decision-making. I'm doing an MSc in health psychology, focusing specifically on shared decision-making.

I also use it in my personal life. I carefully guide my mental health professionals through the Open Talk model discussed later in this chapter, giving them hints as to what they should be asking or saying next. I've got sneaky ways of getting my views and preferences considered, and I'm used to asking, 'How much say do I have in this decision?' to remind my physical and mental health professionals that certain things are ultimately down to me.

But here's the thing: I shouldn't have to. People shouldn't have to spend ten years obsessed with shared decision-making to be involved in decisions about their own lives. When we created Open Talk, my personal experience made the project feel of particular importance. Children and young people in mental health services get a bad deal. A lot of people don't see the value of listening to children. A lot of people also don't see the value of listening to people enveloped in mental illness. CAMHS patients get a double whammy. My time in CAMHS was pretty traumatic. I can't help but think that if I had experienced a shared decision-making approach, it might have cushioned the blow. It is my hope and belief that Open Talk begins to give professionals the skills to provide that metaphorical cushion for the CAMHS patients of today.

Shared decision-making

Shared decision-making (SDM) is at the heart of person-centred care, where patients are partners in planning, developing and assessing care to make sure it is most appropriate for their needs, lives and preferences (Health Foundation, 2012; Health Foundation, 2014a; Health Foundation, 2014b). It means giving equal weight to the knowledge, views and expertise of patients alongside professional or scientific knowledge (NHS England, 2018). The knowledge and expertise young people can bring includes about their needs and how care and support will fit with their everyday lives, their values, goals, and what risks and benefits they are willing to accept and what they are willing to trade off (Health Foundation, 2012; Health Foundation, 2014a; Health Foundation, 2014b). Patients' values, preferences and knowledge are vital for SDM because research shows there is a gap between what patients want and what professionals think they want, and far too many decisions are made in ignorance because they do not take account of patient preferences (Mulley et al, 2012). All decisions have risks, benefits, and trade-offs, and professionals cannot recommend the right treatment without knowing how the patient values these trade-offs (Mulley et al, 2012).

SDM is therefore an ethical imperative in mental health where people have the right to make informed choices about what happens to their bodies and minds (Drake and Deegan, 2009; Drake et al, 2010). This may be particularly important as mental health decisions are rarely clear-cut and often involve complex trade-offs, which are (arguably) best evaluated and assessed by people themselves (Drake et al, 2010). As Drake et al suggest:

> Instead of isolating people in their experience of suffering and resilience, shared decision-making is about sharing and collaborating as partners with medical practitioners. (2010, p 9)

Shared decision-making in mental health inpatient units

The following sections explore the constraints on SDM identified during an ethnographic study (Martin, 2019). The study, in two mental health inpatient units in England, explored how young people (aged 13–17) and staff understood and experienced SDM; and the structures, mechanisms, contexts and relationships that enabled or constrained decision-making.

SDM means bringing the knowledge, values and expertise of young people into decision-making processes, alongside professional knowledge and evidence. This, therefore, requires that the young person and their testimony – their inner self – is heard, involved and influential. However, the research revealed that these are the very things that are, in many ways, routinely constrained or denied within the material environment, systems and routines in inpatient units. The following sections explore some of the key issues and challenges that can affect and constrain young people's ability to be involved in decisions and the ability of staff to involve them.

Amy's reflections

When I was unwell, I spent a lot of time in mental health wards. Initially I was resigned to having every decision taken out of my hands. Like all good teenagers, I ended up rebelling. One day, a staff member poured me a glass of squash absent-mindedly, without asking which flavour I would prefer. It was the straw that broke the camel's back. I had what the staff termed as one of my 'tantrums' – resulting in me being restrained and injected with sedatives. They couldn't see why I was so bothered about a glass of squash, and I didn't know how to understand or verbalise it myself. Looking back, I realise that when the big decisions are out of your hands, the little ones really do matter. Staff routinely taking small decisions out of my hands with the best of intentions may have actually contributed to my disordered behaviour. I am sure that the professionals had no idea of the impact of small decisions on me, my identity and my ability to get better. This is why the SDM matters and needs to be integrated into the practice of all staff, focusing on all decisions.

The choice that limits all others

> 'They didn't give me a choice. They just went, "No, we're ringing your parents now or you're going to get an ambulance, that's it," and um, I didn't even know why I was coming here at the hospital. They said, "You've got to get in a car," and I was confused why I've got to get in a car and they took me here so I didn't know.' Rebecca, young person

Similarly to other young people in the unit, Rebecca described her admission as being uncertain and disorientating. Young people remembered having little real involvement in the decision or process of being admitted, or not even knowing where they were going. Their admission began with a lack of choice or control. The significant majority of young people felt their admission was primarily based on the concerns of others about the risks they posed rather than on their own desire to seek help and support, or on their own constructions of their difficulties. Those who did agree to being admitted did so either to 'relieve the burden' on their families, or as a last resort based on an expectation of intensive therapy – yet were deeply let down when their expectations were not met. As Dan describes, this initial lack of choice set the context that, for him, limited all other choices:

'Umm … The day that they sent me here, I kind of accepted that like, well, I don't really have a choice, like I'm gonna be sent here anyway.' Dan, young person

For some young people, their admission into the inpatient unit was also their first contact with any form of mental health service, as they were admitted after having their first mental health crisis. They were either sectioned or admitted with the consent of their parents. They described having (or remembering) little or no involvement in the decision-making process or little explanation about what was happening to them. Some described being aware of the challenges caused by their mental health crisis (of already being confused and distressed) and understood the need for others to be involved in making the decision for them to be admitted. However, they described that not having involvement or explanation was frightening, confusing and disorientated them even further.

Therefore, young people's experience or perception of having no choice began before and during admission, meaning that from their initial entrance into the unit they felt disempowered. Even those who had some level of involvement in admission decisions felt as if they had no real choice, as they agreed to admission as the last resort for help or because they did not want to be a burden on their families. It is easy to imagine how traumatic and confusing this could be, particularly for a young person who would normally be beginning to reach out for independence, and were instead experiencing exclusion from such an important decision.

Young people were suddenly in a new and strange environment, away from family and friends they knew and trusted, and places that felt familiar, to a place some understood as being based on stereotypes of asylums or prisons. This made them uncertain, suspicious and unsettled. The journey and the arrival into a strange, unknown environment meant young people were removed from their known points of reference – they were physically dislocated and out of place. These experiences communicated that they had no real choice, and being in the unit therefore began with a lack of expectation of having any choice or control.

Time and talk as trust

> 'Even the first day, staff were really nice, funny ... Yeah, they made it like more homely, because they would sit down and they'd play games. They was funny. They would like crack jokes with me and stuff, come sit with you while you're watching TV. Dunno, they was just like older brothers and sisters [laughs].' Dan, young person

Most young people described positive, caring relationships with staff as being one of the most critical factors in feeling cared for, heard and understood. When time equalled care, it consisted of being able to interact in normal, human ways (as they would expect to do with people they lived with intimately outside hospital) and have conversations about seemingly insignificant things, as well as about their treatment and care. They valued simple things, such as just being able to spend time talking or doing things together, talking about day-to-day topics rather than just conversations about their care, as well as humour and warmth. For young people, there was a great need for normal mutual exchange of the kind they would expect between friends and family they trusted. This helped them to feel like a person rather than a patient, as someone who was trusted as well as trusting, and known rather than just observed.

The time and space to have discussions about their care and support enabled young people to develop trust in the professionals. Discussion and deliberation were usually the most important aspects of decision-making for young people, because this made them feel heard, seen and known. In addition to influencing the outcome of a decision, talking openly and frankly about the different options or restrictions enabled young people to understand and learn how to make decisions. As Jimena explained:

> 'If you knew everything and like, had all of the decisions, and the discussions, just everything was out there on the table ... And you work through it together, you'd be more respecting and allowing and

"okay, she knows what she's talking about. I'm going to trust her that she will help me.'" Jimena, young person

---

Amy's reflections

I owe my life to some of the staff who have worked with me over the years. I don't refer to keeping me physically safe – that bit is relatively easy. Building trust, having someone to talk to, and being seen as a human being was what allowed me to leave mental health services and create a successful and fulfilling life.

However, while time and talk with staff was highly valued, this was also limited, restricted and undermined by the many processes of observation and assessment.

Observations over voice

Young people valued time and deliberation with staff which made them feel known, heard, trusted and trusting, yet the inpatient units were dominated by the management of risk, and practices and processes designed to monitor and observe actions and behaviours and the risks young people were deemed to pose or potentially pose. This was in strong contradiction to the things young people (and many of the staff) valued and hoped for, such as time, trust and normal human interactions.

This meant young people were concerned about being assessed or judged on their visible actions and behaviours, rather than their real underlying feelings or motivations. Many felt that staff could not possibly know, through observations, how they were feeling physically or emotionally, which is of course completely correct. Without asking, how could staff understand a patient's thoughts and feelings? They felt that only they could tell staff about their physical and emotional experience and state, yet felt observations took precedence over their experience:

> 'Like, no matter how much they're trained and no matter how much they try, the professionals don't

know what's going on in your head as well as you do. Your body knows everything about what's going on.' Siobhan, young person

For Robert, he came to believe the views of others over his own feelings:

'[Staff say] "Oh, I've seen an improvement in his mood so..." But that could be anything; that could be like some ... something at home ... it might be nothing to do with therapy. So it would just be, I don't know, "I've seen this happen so he must be better." I thought, "Well, I don't feel better but they're saying I must be better," I was just thinking, "Well, it must be just like the normal way people feel, then. Everyone must feel like this, then." But then it took me a long time to realise not everyone's like this.' Robert, young person

---

Amy's reflections

When I was 16, I ordered my notes from my time on the ward. I compared them to my carefully kept and dated diary entries. Sometimes staff seemed to have got the wrong end of the stick. Other times we seemed to be on two different planets. I got upset and frustrated as I read through two different versions of my past. I spent hours thinking 'if only they had told me that at the time', or 'God, I wish they had asked me'. Observations of me didn't express how I was thinking and feeling and yet there it was, in black and white. My notes were wrong because they took professional experience as more important than my personal feelings. There are some things only I knew, and yet observation seemed to make staff put words in my mouth.

Young people felt as if their bodily appearances and actions, as observed by staff, took precedence over their expression of their physical and emotional feelings, experiences and states. This left some feeling as if they were being guarded and supervised, which in turn led them to feel silenced and as if their views carried little weight.

Choice or best interests?

SDM was also a term often used to actually describe decisions made in young people's best interests. When staff talked about discussing decisions with young people, they often described listening to young people's views, which they then used to inform their decision, rather than young people having influence or involvement in negotiating or deliberating what the best option might be. As Siobhan and others explained, this felt as if they were being informed rather than involved:

> 'It was more like "this is a worry so this is what we're going to do", rather than "this is a worry, what do you think?"' Siobhan, young person

During interviews staff were asked to describe examples of how they involved young people in decisions or to think of a time when they thought they had done so particularly well. When describing their approach, staff used language such as "I weighed up…", "I thought about…" Many concluded that their examples were less collaborative than they had thought. Staff described *thinking* through the key steps of making a decision internally or with colleagues – thinking about options, weighing up risks and benefits, and thinking about young people's views. While they were thoughtful with regard to young people, they were often not explicitly involving them in the process. Arguably, this 'shared decision-making behind closed doors' could not really be of benefit to the patient or the professionals, with more realistic plans being reliant on all key stakeholders' input.

As Sara, a psychiatrist, described, the level of influence she allowed young people to have depended on how invested she was in a particular option. If she believed firmly in one, she would inform young people why that was the best one. If she did not have a preference, *then* she would give that choice to them:

'I tend to set the scene first of all very clearly that we're the, we're the staff, we're the doctors. We've got some understanding of the condition that they have. Umm, I tend to give quite clear advice with the reasons behind and the pros and cons. If there are things which it really doesn't matter which way it goes, then I'm, you know, say, you know... Obviously include people very much in those decisions and say, it really doesn't matter and you can think it through and either one is fine. But if there's one where it really do—... Where I really do think one option is better than the other, then I'll be very clear about that. Yes, yeah. I'd explain to them why I've come to that decision, and that is about weighing up pros and cons of the different things. So I'd, I'd do that, but I'd explain how I'd weighed it up.' Sara, psychiatrist

When young people were given information, this was often to make them understand why staff had made a certain decision, rather than to give them choice or influence. For example, some young people described talking to a pharmacist about their medication, but this was often after they had been prescribed the medication to enable them to understand why they were on it.

'I really think it's very important for them to talk to us because it just, it just helps a lot more when you know what's going to happen. It allows you to prepare for it and act in a certain way, like ... whereas, if you're not told the information, you don't know what's going to happen and you start, I don't know, you start actually then making up certain thoughts of what's going to happen and you start thinking a lot more about it. A lot more stress, basically. Whereas if you're told, you know what's going to happen, and you're much more accepting of it.' Hamza, young person

Some staff avoided sharing information about the risks and side effects of medications because they felt it would make young people refuse to take it. The provision or withholding of information was at times used as a tool to conceal, convince and coerce, rather than to share knowledge, inform and empower young people in their thinking and deliberating. There were therefore contradictions and conflict in the teams between those who believed information was there to convince or persuade young people to accept staff decisions and those who saw information as a right to empower and inform them (including the right to refuse).

> 'Because mental health, it's not the same as physical health, basically, and I think, because mental health ... there's a lot of individualism and a lot of your say. A lot of effect that it has ... a lot of it depends on you.'
> Hamza, young person

Being a knower and a decision maker

SDM was also undermined by a lack of trust in young people's views. Young people felt they were not believed owing to assumptions about the diagnostic label they had been given. Jaime and Emily both described how they often experienced their expressions, actions or preferences being explained as a symptom of their eating disorder. Young people were often doubted based on assumptions about their diagnosis – as if certain diagnoses, such as borderline personality disorder (BPD) or eating disorders, equated to their views being less reliable. Some felt they were doubted due to their age or for how they acted. Others felt their views were given less weight due to how they behaved, particularly if they were seen by others as difficult or challenging:

> 'Because I feel sometimes the staff, like ... I misbehave quite a lot, but then they don't take me as seriously as they take some of the other people.'
> Louise, young person

Many young people felt that their views were taken less seriously owing to the way in which they expressed them, as if distress or visible expressions of emotion made their views less real or reliable:

> 'If you say something and they don't agree with you, that doesn't mean they can't help you in another way. But then they will say some, like "this isn't a hotel, this is a hospital, just accept the treatment you've been given."' Asif, young person

Young people described how their views were also doubted or undermined if they did not agree with staff. Asif described how his refusal to take medication was seen as a refusal of help or as proof of his lack of capacity. Asif had strong views about medication and did not want it take it due to his faith. He expressed deep concerns about the impact on his body and wanted to know what impact the medications would have. However, he said his reasons for refusal were dismissed as being unfounded, as if he were being difficult and refusing treatment because he was too unwell to make a decision, rather than refusing a *form of treatment*. He said he was not refusing treatment, but he was resistant to taking medication. Refusal or disagreement were often seen as typical teenage behaviour rather than valid differences of opinion. Young people's reasons for resistance were constructed as invalid or immature, as if they should just passively comply with adult authority. For example, they were often told "you have to understand…". This led young people to feel dismissed, unheard or increasingly frustrated, which in turn affected how they acted and added further 'proof' of their 'volatility'.

While many staff wanted to believe in and trust young people, their decision to trust (or how much to trust) young people's views (or not) could have very real consequences and could entail high levels of risk, distress or harm. They were aware that the decisions they made, such as whether to let young people have their shoelaces or not, could have significant consequences.

They were therefore very vigilant about whether they could trust young people's views and the weight of thinking 'but what if…' For example, staff described memories of young people harming themselves in the past, as well as anticipation of the possible harm to come if they trusted young people and got it wrong. Many staff described how, when considering a decision that would affect a young person, they would think about whether they could defend their decision in a court of law if someone came to harm. This could make staff err on the side of caution rather than trust young people.

I'm not a decision maker

Many young people did not see themselves as decision makers and felt they could not or should not be involved in decision-making. Some young people felt they were unable to make decisions due to their mental health difficulties or distress. They felt their mental health difficulties had more agency and influence over decision-making than they did. Jaime, a young woman, felt that if she got involved in decision-making it "would probably be the illness" talking and so any expression of preference "wouldn't be for the right reason". Other young people, like Melissa, felt that "if you're mentally ill, you don't really know what's going on around you". The way she saw her distress made her feel powerless and as if others (her parents or professionals) should make decisions for her.

Similarly, other young people doubted their own ability to be involved due to their age. Many assumed that they could not be involved in decisions because they were young (this included 16- and 17-year-olds) or felt they should defer to professionals:

> 'Because the psychiatrist said it would be good and
> I was like, well they're the professional.' Siobhan,
> young person

They perceived that they were making decisions with the setting in its entirety, with its powerful systems and structures, not just with individual staff, and therefore felt overwhelmed and powerless. They could not see how they could have any influence on what was happening around them. Their self-image was one of passivity and powerlessness, and they were resigned to not being involved in decisions or discussions that affected them, in the face of the many constraints of their environment.

Discussion

SDM is not merely a moment or a one-off event. Whether young people feel heard and able to be involved in decisions – and whether staff have any real opportunity to involve young people in meaningful decisions – are heavily influenced and constrained by the many practices and constraints within inpatient units. These practices and constraints undermine the core elements of SDM. Young people's views and the time, talk and trust they need to feel heard are outweighed by routines, observations, assessments and processes driven by risk.

To ensure SDM becomes more explicit, many changes are need in the processes and systems in inpatient units to enable staff to meaningfully involve young people and to enable young people to have more freedom and choice. SDM and the extent to which young people are able to be heard and influential is not merely determined by the moments in which staff are trying to involved them in decisions – it is affected by all of their experiences of admission into and being in the unit. Young people need to be more involved in decisions about their admission (or at least, acknowledgement and reflection on the impact on their lack of choice). Similarly, they need to be more involved in their day-to-day care and processes of making meaning of their feelings and experiences, rather than distant observations and record-keeping. Systems and processes need to be radically redesigned to support real choice, rather than be dominated by the management of risk. The observations suggest a system in need of change, with staff feeling burdened with important decisions, and young people feeling unheard or unimportant. Further research is needed to identify what differences these changes make to how young people see themselves as decision makers and the experiences of staff in trying to involve young people.

Amy's reflections

Recovery is more than a game of chess played by others, on the patient's behalf. Having been very unwell and achieved a complete recovery, I know that getting better is hard work. However, without understanding what is happening and why, being involved in thinking through options and having values heard and understood, most of us would be unlikely to do whatever we were told without a fuss. The issues in this chapter are not intended to point blame at mental health professionals. Instead, they are thinking and talking points, and a reminder of the need to stand in the patient's shoes and ask the question, 'How would I react to my choices being made in this way?'

Supporting shared decision-making in mental health

Significant changes are needed within services to overcome the constraints on SDM. Open and explicit conversations with young people are vital in ensuring young people are heard and understood. While tools do not do SDM in and of themselves, they can assist with elements of the decision-making process as, for example, they can help to balance power, make SDM more tangible for young people, and increase their sense of control (Wolpert et al, 2014). There are a small but increasing number of tools to assist and support SDM in young people's mental health services. In a review of tools and approaches to support SDM in children and young people's mental health, 22 records were identified and grouped under six types of approach, which included therapeutic techniques, decision aids, psycho-educational information, action planning or goal setting, discussion prompts, and approaches that mobilised patients to engage (Hayes et al, 2018). However, of the 22 identified, 12 of these were aimed at parents rather than children and young people (Hayes et al, 2018).

The Open Talk model (Martin, 2017) was co-produced with young people to build on Makoul and Clayman (2006) and Wolpert et al (2014) to encourage open deliberation with young people to ensure their views and preferences are at the heart of decisions that affect them. The model has been used to facilitate training and reflective practice with staff working in CAMHS to support them to explore how to make decision-making more open and explicit, particularly in more challenging scenarios

Figure 1.1: The Open Talk model

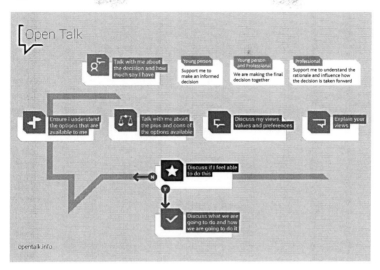

Source: Martin (2017)

(for example, where the young person has not chosen to access support or where there is disagreement).

The Open Talk model has three key stages: setting up the conversation with the young person; the middle stages of deliberation and negotiation; and the end stages to clarify what has been decided and what the next steps are.

Beginning stage: setting up the conversation

Young people are often unclear about what decisions they can be involved in, assume they do not have any influence, or assume they will be informed about what decisions have been made about them by others. The first stage of the model is therefore to ensure young people know they are involved and how much influence they have.

Talk with me about the decision and how much say I have:
Support me to know:

• that there is a decision to make;

- what the decision is about;
- how much influence I have in the decision.

Middle stages: thinking and deliberating together

The middle stages should enable the young person and professional to both contribute to thinking about what options and possibilities there are, their pros and cons, and how these fit with the young person's goals, views, values and circumstances.

Ensure I understand the options available to me:
- Ask me what options I think there are.
- Talk with me about what options you think I have. This may include deciding to do nothing.
- Explore what each option entails.
- Explore what I have already tried, what has and hasn't worked, and whether I want to revisit these again.
- Remember to be open to discussing all options, even if you may not be able to support me with these – I need to explore them all to understand what will and won't work for me and why.

Talk with me about the pros and cons of the options:
- Support me to think through and weigh up the pros and cons of each option.
- Consider whether there is information to help me to understand the pros and cons, for example is there an evidence base?
- Be open to discussing all the pros and cons – I need to explore them all to understand what will and won't work for me and why.
- Explore what we disagree and agree about and why.

Discuss my views, values and preferences:
- Talk with me about how I feel about the different options, their pros and cons, their impact and what is important to me.
- Explore any worries or concerns I have.
- Explore what I think others in my life might think and feel about the different options, and how I feel this could influence my decision.

- Remember that a whole list of pros might be outweighed by one con, if that is the thing that's most important to me.

Explain your views:
- Explain what you think is the best option for me, based on what you know about me, research evidence, your professional experience, and what has (and hasn't) worked for other young people – be careful not to 'recommend' one 'option'.
- Consider that your preferred option might not be what is best for me or what I feel able to do.
- If there are options you cannot support explain why, acknowledge my views and talk with me about what we can do together.

Discuss if I feel able to do this:
- Clarify how able I feel to do this. This might be different from what I think is the best option.
- Talk with me about how I could do this and what support I might need.
- If I don't think I can do this, we may need to revisit earlier options.

End stages: summarising and putting it into action

Discuss what we are going to do and how we are going to do it:
Check and clarify my understanding about what decision has been made and why:

- Plan with me how I will put this into practice, and what support I may need.
- Check if it would be helpful to record our discussion and decision, and what format of record-keeping would be best for me.
- Agree when we will reflect on and review the decision.
- Remember this may include the fact that we cannot reach a decision yet or that we can clearly acknowledge we disagree.

Summary

SDM in mental health services is significantly constrained by systems and processes of services privileging the management of risk over the views and choices of young people. SDM is more than a transactional one-off moment or event. It is enabled or constrained by young people's experiences of admission into and within inpatient services, and relationships, interactions and systems. Further research is needed to identify how to overcome these constraints to enhance practices that focus on respecting the views of young people, and the places, people and relationships they know and trust. This should not just be in moments of decision-making, but in all interactions, practices and systems within mental healthcare and support.

Note

[1] www.health.org.uk/improvement-projects/shared-decision-making-in-child-and-adolescent-mental-health-care

References

Drake, R.E. and Deegan, P.E. (2009) Shared decision making is an ethical imperative. *Psychiatric Services*, 60 (8), p 1007.

Drake, R.E., Deegan, P.E. and Rapp, C. (2010) The promise of shared decision making in mental health. *Psychiatric Rehabilitation Journal*, 34 (1), pp 7–13.

Hayes, C., Simmons, M., Simons, C. and Hopwood, M. (2018) Evaluating effectiveness in adolescent mental health inpatient units: A systematic review. *International Journal of Mental Health Nursing*, 27 (2), pp 498–513.

Health Foundation (2012) *Helping people share decisions: A review of evidence considering whether shared decision making is worthwhile.* London: The Health Foundation.

Health Foundation (2014a) *Helping measure person-centred care.* London: The Health Foundation.

Health Foundation (2014b) *Person-centred care: from ideas to action. Bringing together the evidence on shared decision making and self-management support.* London: The Health Foundation.

Makoul, G. and Clayman, M. (2006) An integrative model of shared decision-making in medical encounters. *Patient Education and Counseling*, 60 (3), pp 301–12.

Martin, K. (2017) *Open Talk model of shared decision-making* [online]. Available from: https://goals-in-therapy.com/2020/05/22/open-talk-decision-making-with-young-people-in-mental-health/

Martin, K. (2019) A critical realist study of shared decision-making in young people's mental health inpatient units. PhD thesis, University College London, London.

Mulley, A., Trimble, C. and Elwyn, G. (2012). *Patients' preferences matter: Stop the silent misdiagnosis.* London: The King's Fund. Available from: https://www.kingsfund.org.uk/publications/patients-preferences-matter

NHS England (2018) *Shared decision-making.* Available from: www.england.nhs.uk/shared-decision-making/about/ [Last accessed: 23rd September].

Wolpert, M., Hoffman, J., Abrines, N., Feltham, A., Baird, L., Law, D., Martin, K., Constable, A. and Hopkins, K. (2014) *Closing the gap: Shared decision making in CAMHS: Final report for closing the gap through changing relationships.* London: The Health Foundation.

2

Disabled young people's participation in end-of-life decisions

Zoe Picton-Howell

Introduction

This chapter draws on my academic research and lived experience as mum to Adam. My research explored how UK paediatricians make end-of-life decisions for disabled children and young people, and how they use, or choose not to use the law and professional guidance in those decisions (Picton-Howell, 2018). Adam lived with severe physical impairment. He was educationally bright. He spent, in total, eight years of his life in hospital, meaning so did I. Adam acquired severe cerebral palsy at birth in 2000 and developed significant complex health problems. He died from sepsis in 2015.

Background

Adam's healthcare experience was extensive; with care in seven tertiary,[1] district[2] and specialist children's hospitals across the UK. He was treated by health professionals with expertise in a broad range of health conditions. He had daily contact with NHS staff on almost every day of his life.

Over the years, I noticed differences in how health professionals engaged with Adam. Nurses, therapists and doctors who were not paediatricians (doctors specialising in the treatment of children and young people), for example general practitioners, tended to engage with Adam, including him in decisions, without difficulty. In contrast, while some paediatricians engaged with him, many did not, assuming, based on Adam's physical impairment and health problems, that he was unable to communicate or understand. I noticed that female and younger paediatricians were more likely to engage with Adam, and male and older paediatricians were less likely to do so.

The context of Adam's life more generally is perhaps relevant here. He attended mainstream school and was always at the top end of the ability range educationally for his age. He blogged and wrote poetry and as a teenager was regularly commissioned to write by the NHS nationally and by charities. He won multiple national and international awards for his writing and advocacy. He was interviewed by regional and national media. What perhaps surprised me most is that some paediatricians, even when they were told all this by me or their colleagues, still insisted Adam could not understand or communicate.

Adam's main method of communication was blinking. At its most simple, he would blink for 'yes' and give an obvious stare for 'no', but he developed sophisticated methods enabling him to discuss complex ideas. He also spelt out words using a spelling chart and when older used an electronic 'voice'. One thing that intrigued me was that the only people who ever questioned Adam's abilities were some paediatricians. He conversed without problem with his teachers and classmates. He chatted to friends, family and neighbours, but he also had no difficulty communicating with people on meeting them for the first time. He chatted with shop assistants and successfully purchased items; he often chatted to authors when he visited the local annual book festival and he gave a talk to members of the Scottish Parliament. He was interviewed by journalists several times, including just months before his death when he was the face of NHS England's Change Day campaign encouraging health professionals to engage with children and young people.

Although Adam's methods of communication were unusual, they were clear and quick and easy to learn. It is difficult not to conclude that Adam was excluded from participating by some paediatricians not because Adam *could* not communicate with them, but because those paediatricians *would* not communicate with him.

The assumptions some paediatricians made about Adam, despite clear evidence of his obvious ability to understand and communicate, inspired me as an academic and a lawyer to embark on a PhD exploring which factors UK paediatricians consider and the weight they put on them when making decisions for disabled children and young people. One of the factors I asked paediatricians about was the weight they put on a child or young person's views of the treatment he or she should or should not receive. This chapter draws on findings from that study and wider research.

I start by reviewing the legal and professional obligations on UK doctors to promote children and young people's participation in decisions about their healthcare. I then present what the UK paediatricians said in my study about severely disabled children and young people participating in potentially end-of-life treatment decisions. I end with some recommendations to improve young people's participation in healthcare decisions.

My study considered children from the age of two years old to young people up to the age of 18. However, much of what the paediatricians said is also relevant to young people up to the age of 25 and in some cases even older. The paediatricians in my study were reflecting on their use of the law. As will be seen, there are significant changes in the law when a young person reaches 16. For conciseness, unless the context makes it necessary, for the rest of this chapter the term 'young person' or 'young people' is used to include 'child' or 'children'.

Although my study looked at paediatricians, its findings and Adam's experiences are relevant to all health professionals working with young people, because of the influential role played by health professionals in many disabled young people's lives.

What is participation according to law and professional guidance?

In this chapter my focus is young people's participation in decisions about their own healthcare, rather than participation in wider strategic decisions. It should, however, be noted that rights discussed in this chapter also apply to those wider decisions.[3]

A right for young people to participate is found in Article 12 of the United Nation's Convention of the Rights of the Child (UNCRC).[4] Before looking at the substance of this right, it worth first considering the status of the UNCRC within the UK to help understand its impact. Although ratified[5] by the UK in 1991[6] the UNCRC has not yet[7] been incorporated into UK domestic law.[8] This makes enforcement within the UK difficult, as a young person has no clear legal remedy. However, ratification short of incorporation still imposes obligations on the UK government to ensure young people's UNCRC rights are fulfilled. One mechanism used is for UNCRC rights to be echoed or cited in domestic legislation, but this tends to be rather piecemeal.[9] Another mechanism is the reporting obligations the UNCRC places on states to periodically[10] report to the UNCRC Committee made up of internationally recognised independent experts, on the steps being taken by the state to fulfil their UNCRC obligations.[11] Civil society, including voluntary organisations, academics and those working directly with young people also submit a parallel report.[12] The reports can be found on the UN Human Rights Commission website and make interesting, if somewhat depressing, reading.[13] In theory, having to report periodically to the UNCRC Committee should put international pressure on the UK government to ensure UNCRC rights are met. However, reading the civil society reports suggests improvements in fulfilling young people's rights are slow. The UK could opt into further UNCRC mechanisms to help fulfil UNCRC rights, for example allowing young people to take complaints directly to the UNCRC Committee or allowing the UNCRC to carry out inquiries within the UK. The UK government has not taken up these options.

Irrespective of these barriers to fulfilment, the UNCRC Committee make clear that Article 12 imposes a legal obligation on governments to ensure young people can participate in decisions that impact on their lives.[14] If legal mechanisms are not doing this effectively, arguably educating staff including health professionals working with young people is an important step in raising awareness of young people's UNCRC rights. Indeed, in their latest periodic report to the UNCRC Committee, the UK government recognise this and report education on the UNCRC as being a '*key element*' of the training provided to all staff working with young people (UN, 2015, emphasis added).[15] Despite this assertion and similar claims in earlier UK periodic reports, all 33 paediatricians in my study reported never having received education or training in the UNCRC, making them unlikely to act in ways that ensure young people's rights are fulfilled.

A detailed explanation of what Article 12 requires is found in General Comment 12 (GC12) issued by the UNCRC Committee (UN, 2009).[16] General Comments issued by UN Committees on particular articles or themes act as detailed guides, expanding on a treaty article's meaning and suggesting how best to ensure its fulfilment.

GC12 makes clear that Article 12 places a legal obligation on states to ensure all young people, capable of forming their own views, have the right to express those views freely and for them to be given due weight according to the young person's age and maturity.[17] GC12 makes clear that simply listening to a young person is not sufficient; their views have to be seriously considered.[18] It confirms that Article 12 creates not just a right for a young person to take part in decisions about their own healthcare but also wider policy and strategic decisions.[19] It is also worthy of note, that Article 12 includes the right not to take part in the decision-making process.[20]

Rights to participate in domestic law

The participation rights of young people in England and Wales[21] aged 16 and above are also protected by the Mental Capacity Act 2005 (MCA). This provides a legal framework aimed at empowering people to make decisions for themselves as far as they are able. It also puts in place mechanisms enabling people to plan ahead to a time when they may not have capacity, perhaps through ill health or impairment. The MCA has a Code of Practice[22] which all health professionals are obliged to follow. Five key principles underpin the MCA;[23] (i) a presumption of capacity; (ii) individuals must be supported to make their own decisions; (iii) people have a right to make unwise decisions; (iv) anything done for or on behalf of someone who lacks mental capacity must be done in their best interests; (v) the least restrictive option should be taken, meaning the option which interferes least with the individuals' rights. There is not space in this chapter to discuss the MCA in detail, but it is not a statute without its critics. The House of Lords Select Committee on the MCA found both a lack of awareness and a lack of understanding of the MCA. It concluded:

> The general lack of awareness of the provisions of the Act has allowed prevailing professional practices to continue unchallenged, and allowed decision-making to be dominated by professionals. (House of Lords, 2014a, p 8, para 6)

The presumption of capacity was particularly poorly understood. Under the MCA 'a person is not to be treated as unable to make a decision unless all practicable steps to help him to do so have been taken to do so without success'.[24] The House of Lords found this was 'rare in practice', with the MCA being used as a framework to make decisions *for* a person, 'rather than encouraging or maximising their participation in the decision making' (House of Lords, 2014a, p 41, para 79).

In addition to the MCA, in England and Wales, the Family Law Reform Act 1969,[25] also creates a presumption that a 16- or 17-year-old is competent to consent to medical treatment and therefore competent to actively participate in decisions about their healthcare. But once again, the problem arises both of health professionals being aware of the legislation and implementing it correctly. As will be seen later in this chapter, paediatricians in my study suggested that for disabled young people, this presumption tends to be reversed, with a presumption being made that a disabled young person is not competent to be involved in decisions about their own healthcare. Adam's experience suggested that this happens even in the face of clear evidence of a young person's competence.

For young people under the age of 16, the situation is perhaps more difficult as there is no statutory right or statutory Code of Practice setting out their right to participate. Instead they have to rely on what lawyers call 'Common Law', that is, law derived mainly from decisions of the courts and arguably far less accessible than statutes.

Many health professionals will have heard of the English common law Gillick Principle. This is used to assess whether a young person is 'Gillick competent', 'capable of making a reasonable assessment of the advantages of the treatment proposed'.[26] Like the UNCRC and MCA, Gillick competence is often poorly understood and applied by health professionals. It is important to understand that a young person is not either Gillick competent or not Gillick competent. A young person may be competent to make some decisions but not others, or to make a decision in some circumstances but not others. The age and stage at which a young person becomes Gillick competent in relation to a decision will also vary from young person to young person.

Gillick competence, of course, deals with consenting to treatment, rather than participation. It is important to remember that while Gillick competence can certainly be evidence that a young person is fully able to participate in a decision and indeed make it, lack of Gillick competence must not be taken as evidence that a young person is unable to participate at all. As was seen from Article 12 UNCRC, all young people who wish to do so should legally be supported to participate in healthcare decisions *as far as they are able*.

Having established what the law says about young people's participation, this chapter now considers what doctors' guidance says.

What does doctors' guidance say about young people's participation?

Medical doctors working in the UK have a professional obligation to encourage young people's participation in decisions about their healthcare (General Medical Council (GMC), 2018).

GMC[27] 0–18, which all UK-based doctors must follow, tells doctors they *must* respect young people's views (GMC, 2018) calling this an 'overriding duty'.[28]

GMC 0–18 gives examples of how participation can be facilitated:

> (d) explain things using language or other forms of communication they can understand; (e) consider how you and they use non-verbal communication... (f) give them the opportunities to ask questions, and answer them honestly and to the best of your ability.[29]

However, GMC 0–18 arguably gives doctors too much leeway to exclude a young person from decisions, without first doing as much as possible to facilitate involvement. GMC 0–18 makes clear that doctors do not have to respect a young person's rights in circumstances beyond the doctor's control.[30] This is a particular risk for disabled young people, as will be discussed later.

While acknowledging that there will be circumstances when a young person cannot participate, for example if he or she is too young; too ill; or lacks the ability to understand the decision, there will still be many circumstances when a young person can participate if properly supported. Moreover, although alternative communication methods are mentioned there is no obligation for a doctor to use them. As Adam's experience showed, young people who can participate using alternative communication methods can be excluded from participating.

GMC 0–18 applies to all child healthcare. Doctors also have guidance dealing with care at the end of a young person's life, which also touches on young people's participation in these decisions. This is now discussed because the paediatricians in my study particularly focused on end-of-life decisions.

Guidance is provided by both medical royal colleges[31] and the National Institute for Health and Care Excellence (NICE).[32] Unlike guidance from the GMC, doctors are not obliged to follow this guidance. However, this guidance is seen as best practice and failing to follow it without good reason may be evidence of poor practice if problems arise.

The Royal College of Paediatrics and Child Health issued guidance in 2015 (Larcher et al, 2015). It gives a comprehensive account of both the law and ethical principles a paediatrician should follow when making end-of-life decisions. However, while generally comprehensive, it says little about the young person's role:

> The professionals' second duty[33] is to respect patients' right to make their own informed choices (autonomy). They should respect patients' rights to as much self-determination as they are capable, and respect their known or ascertainable wishes, beliefs, preferences and values. (para 2.4.1)

NICE also published guidance in 2016 on the care and treatment young people should receive at the end of life (NICE, 2016). Like the RCPCH, the NICE guidance also says little about young people's participation. It does, however, say:

> 1.1.2 Discuss and regularly review with children and young people and their parents or carers how they want to be involved in making decisions about their care, because this varies between individuals, at different times, and depending on what decisions are being made.
> 1.1.3 Explain to children and young people and to their parents or carers that their contribution to decisions about their care is very important, but that they do not have to make decisions alone and the multidisciplinary team will be involved as well.
> 1.1.4 When difficult decisions must be made about end of life care, give children and young people and their parents or carers enough time and opportunities for discussions. (NICE, 2016 para 1.1)

Despite doctors being obliged to follow GMC 0–18 and Larcher et al (2015) and NICE (2016) being seen as best practice, the paediatricians in my study (Picton-Howell, 2018) suggested that guidance may be used less than the drafters, experts in the field including ethicists, lawyers and lay people as well as doctors, anticipate. Only 13 of the 33 paediatricians in my study reported using the RCPCH guidance in place at the time (RCPCH, 2004), and only three paediatricians reported using GMC 0–18. Moreover, those who used either documents, reported doing so to justify their decisions to third parties, such as parents or colleagues, rather than to guide their decisions.

This brief review of the law and doctors' professional guidance suggests that a significant barrier to fulfilling young people's healthcare participation rights is health professionals' poor knowledge and understanding of those rights. Recommendations in this regard are made at the end of this chapter. We now turn to my study which draws upon what the paediatricians said about young people's participation in treatment decisions.

My study

My study (Picton-Howell, 2018) explored UK paediatricians' end-of-life decisions for disabled young people. Thirty-two senior consultants[34] and one specialist registrar[35] completed a survey on the factors they considered; the weight they put on those factors and most importantly for this discussion, whom they included in the decision-making process. It also asked paediatricians about any legal education; their use of professional guidance and assessed how the doctors made sense of the law when making their decisions. The paediatricians also provided information about their personal characteristics, such as age; gender; religious beliefs and personal experience of disability. Nine paediatricians also took part in in-depth semi-structured interviews, discussing in more depth the issues raised in the survey.

Email invitations were sent to 368 paediatricians with a link to the survey. Professional bodies for key paediatric sub-specialisms[36] were also emailed and asked to pass a link to their members. Responses were received from ten paediatric intensive care consultants (30 per cent of participants), nine paediatric neurologists[37] (27 per cent), four general paediatricians[38] (12 per cent) and two respiratory specialists[39] (6 per cent). Two participants (6 per cent) were paediatric endocrine[40] consultants. The remaining participants, all paediatricians, were a metabolic specialist;[41] an oncologist;[42] an emergency specialist;[43] a palliative care specialist;[44] a neonatologist;[45] and a surgeon. Four neurologists; two intensivists; one respiratory consultant; one oncologist and one palliative care consultant took part in the follow-up interviews.

My study included paediatricians who had worked in every UK health region. It also included four paediatricians (12 per cent) who had completed part or all of their medical training abroad and five (15 per cent) who had worked as a qualified doctor abroad. The paediatricians had between 18 and 52 years' experience. Twenty-four (72 per cent) had been qualified for over 25 years.

All the participants were from tertiary hospitals. Most were heads of departments and several influential regionally and some nationally. Twenty paediatricians (60.5 per cent) were male, and nine (27 per cent) female. Four (12 per cent) did not specify their gender. This gender split is in keeping with the ratio of male to female doctors (70%:30%) on the GMC Specialist Register,[46] at the time of my survey (GMC, 2011). All the participants were registered with the RCPCH who reported 43.9 per cent of tertiary consultants being female at the date of my study (RCPCH, 2013), suggesting my participants were disproportionately male. This may be because 35 per cent of the female paediatricians worked part-time (RCPCH, 2014), perhaps giving them less opportunity to complete a survey.

The paediatricians' very senior status also perhaps explains their lack of ethnic diversity. Much is written about 'the snowy white peaks' of the NHS (for example Kline, 2014; Priest et al, 2015) whereby despite the NHS's ethnic diverse workforce, ethnic minorities face significant difficulties in obtaining senior positions. Twenty paediatricians (60.5 per cent) identified themselves as ethnically English, Scottish, Welsh or from Northern Ireland. This perhaps also explains the lack of diversity of religious faith, with 19 paediatricians (57 per cent) describing themselves as Christian, and 13 (39 per cent) as having no religion or faith.

When asked about any personal experience of disability, none of the paediatricians reported having an impairment themselves. A perhaps surprisingly large number did, however, report personal experience of disability, particularly as the parent of a disabled child (six, 18 per cent) or having experience of a close disabled relative, for example a disabled sibling (four, 12 per cent). UK government statistics report 0.8 million (6 per cent) of children in the UK as disabled in 2010/11 (DWP, 2012), using the Equality Act 2010 definition of disability,[47] making 18 per cent of the paediatricians in my study being parents of a disabled child higher than anticipated. I assumed paediatricians whose own child was disabled were drawn to my study because of their personal experience, something the paediatricians to whom this applied confirmed when interviewed.

With just 33 participants, my study was small. It also did not include paediatricians who qualified after 1998. Its strength, however, is that paediatricians who took part not only came from all over the UK, but were also, other than the one specialist registrar, senior consultants in positions of influence. The paediatricians in my study are not presented as representative of paediatricians generally, but rather as the voices of powerful and influential paediatricians from around the UK when end–of–life decisions for disabled young people are being made.

What did the paediatricians say about disabled young people's participation in their decisions?

The paediatricians were given a description of the young people at the focus of my study:

> For the purpose of this study the term 'disabled children' is used to describe children with chronic health conditions and physical and sometimes sensory and cognitive impairments. These children will often have some level of neurological impairment, will often be described as having 'life limiting' conditions, although they will not necessarily be terminally ill. (Picton-Howell, 2018)

The paediatricians were also asked which decisions they found most difficult. All but two reported end–of–life decisions, making these the focus of my study.

The paediatricians were asked two survey questions aimed at exploring how much they encouraged disabled young people to participate in decisions. They were asked: (i) whom they consulted with and (ii) what role the young person played in the decision.

Just three paediatricians (9 per cent) reported including young people in response to question (i). The three did not have any personal or professional characteristics distinguishing them from other participants, so no conclusions can be drawn.

The paediatricians' answers to question (ii) were more enlightening. Eight paediatricians (24 per cent) described the young person as having a central role, and 11 (33 per cent) said the young person would be involved if he or she were old and cognitively able enough. Within these 11, five (15 per cent) gave answers suggesting the paediatrician expected a disabled young person to be able to participate, while, two paediatricians (9 per cent), suggested it was highly unlikely.

Ten further paediatricians (30.3 per cent) suggested a disabled young person would be unable to make a decision or would have very limited involvement in decisions.

While acknowledging that the cognitive ability of young people with severe physical impairment and serious health problems can vary from profound learning difficulties to educationally very able, a concern, and one expressed by paediatricians in my study, is that paediatricians can start with a presumption that a disabled young person will not be able to participate, and therefore they will not even consider the possibility. This seems to echo the findings of the House of Lords Select Committee (House of Lords, 2014a). It was a concern raised by several paediatricians at interview. For example, Participant 29, a senior consultant neurologist, said, talking about his colleagues:

> 'You often find that they have made a mistake, quite honestly and they have grouped the whole set of things together and produced a single score and what they haven't done is looked at the child's islands of development[48] which means that they have got potential.'

Another senior neuro-disability specialist, Participant 24, recalled an incident of a colleague wrongly assuming a disabled young person did not attend school, so would necessarily lack understanding and indeed a quality of life worth preserving.

The split between paediatricians as to the potential for a severely disabled young person to participate is noteworthy. Wilkinson and Truog (2013) describe a 'roster lottery' whereby decisions depend not on the characteristics of the patient, but rather the values of the doctor. A concern echoed by paediatricians in my study. For example, Participant 14 went as far to say that whether a disabled young person lived or died depended on the values and beliefs of the paediatricians treating the young person (which could be different with a different team), not the young person's state of health.

The paediatricians' personal and professional characteristics were used to explore whether paediatricians with particular characteristics seem more likely to encourage young person participation, than paediatricians with different characteristics. You will recall that I had observed with Adam that female and younger paediatricians seemed more likely to encourage his participation. My study unfortunately had low numbers of both female and younger paediatricians. In general terms, the paediatricians' personal and professional characteristics did not seem to impact on their decision-making. There was no suggestion in the data that paediatricians from a particular sub-specialism were either more likely or less likely to view a disabled young person as potentially capable of participating:

Table 2.1: Views on participation by paediatric specialism

Sub-specialism	PICU (%)	Neurology (%)	Other (%)
Young person (YP) plays a central role in decision-making	30	33	14
YP unlikely to be able to be involved	20	33	36
Ability to be involved depends on individual YP's age and ability	30	33	33

Likewise, there was no suggestion of any link between a paediatrician's gender; decade of qualification or adherence or otherwise to a religious faith.

There was, however, a suggestion, which would merit further research in a larger study, that paediatricians who have a personal connection with disability, either as a parent or as a close relative, are perhaps more likely to consider a disabled young person capable of participating in decisions, than paediatricians with no personal connection with disability:

Table 2.2: Views on participation by personal connection with disability

Personal connection with disability	No personal connection (%)	Personal connection (%)	Parent (%)	Other relative (%)
YP plays a central role in decision-making	9	50	50	50
YP unlikely to be able to be involved	39	10	0	36
Ability to be involved depends on individual YP's age and ability	35	30	17	50

Perhaps most importantly, the paediatricians in my study suggested that their colleagues' assessments of a disabled young person's ability to participate had significance beyond just the young person's participation in the decision. They suggested it could be a factor when deciding whether to treat or withhold treatment. Several paediatricians voiced concerns that colleagues withheld or withdrew treatment, based not on clinical factors, such as a young person's diagnosis or prognosis, but on a young person's assumed quality of life, with the assumed ability to participate being key in this assessment. The paediatricians voiced concerns both that this formed part of their colleagues' assessments and as to the accuracy of their colleagues' assessments. The paediatricians therefore suggested that a young person's ability to participate or otherwise in healthcare decisions really is a matter of life or death.

A finding that a doctor's personal characteristics potentially impacts on that doctor's end-of-life decision-making it not surprising. Earlier studies have suggested similar. For example, in their United States-based study, Mebane et al (1999) found significant differences in end-of-life decisions made by white and black doctors. Cuttini et al's (2000) study of 1,235 neonatologists in eight European states, which asked about end-of-life decision-making, found variations in practice both between states and between doctors within a single state, based on the doctor's personal characteristics.

A further finding from my study which is perhaps significant to this whole discussion is of a potential link between a paediatrician's communication style and his or her compliance with law and guidance. When exploring how the paediatricians' make sense of the law in their everyday working lives, the paediatricians were found to fall into two camps. These were *hardliners*, so called because one paediatrician in this camp used this term to describe herself, and *softliners*. The two camps were on a graduating scale rather than binary. Hardliners tended not to consult with colleagues, parents or young people when making decisions. They tended to see themselves as very legally aware, eager to share with me their knowledge of the law. They rejected the possibility that a disabled young person could participate in decisions. They used negative language about parents, for example 'deluded' or 'pathological'. They emphasised the negative aspects of any treatment and tended not to balance these against benefits. Hardliners saw the law as central to their end-of-life decisions. They turned to the law to protect them from prosecution but also expressed fear of it. Hardliners also used heuristics[49] to guide their decisions, for example rules such as a cognitively impaired young person should not receive intensive care. They described making decisions based on a *type* of young person, rather than an *individual*.

In contrast, softliners did not see the law as relevant to their decisions. They consulted widely, involving the young person whenever and however possible, as well as colleagues and parents. They described making decisions based on the individual not a *type* of young person. They spoke about the young person and parents using compassionate language. They emphasised a young person's potential and abilities, as well as the positive aspects of a young person's life, such as the ability to communicate and positive relationships with his or her family and balanced these against the burdens of treatment. They also encouraged parents to advocate for their young person if he or she were unable to communicate a view due to ill health or impairment.

What is perhaps most striking about these two camps is that when their end-of-life decision-making, as described by the paediatricians, is mapped to their professional guidance and the law, it is the softliners, with their wide consultation and balancing the benefits and burdens of treatment for the individual young person, who are making decisions in keeping with the law and guidance. In contrast, the hardliners, while seeing themselves as legally aware, describe decision-making which is out of step with both the law and professional guidance, illustrating that wide participation and good communication are the essence of lawful and ethical end-of-life decision-making.

Conclusions and recommendations

This chapter has highlighted key law and doctors' professional guidance and suggested that a significant barrier to young people's participation in healthcare decisions is health professionals' awareness, understanding and application of that law and professional guidance. The paediatricians in my study also suggested an unwillingness by some paediatricians to accept a disabled young person's rights and ability to participate in decisions. Adam's experience echoed this with key paediatricians refusing to accept his ability to participate, despite all the evidence to the contrary.

My first recommendation is therefore better education and training in law and professional guidance for health professionals, but particularly doctors. It is important that this is provided by experts in the law and, when relevant, disabled people's lives. Indeed, as I saw first-hand with Adam when a training film[50] he made about the UNCRC was used with health professionals, an extremely impactful way to do this is to involve, as far as possible, disabled young people in this training and education.

It was seen earlier that an aim of the MCA is to facilitate long-term planning and ensure a young person's wishes and preferences can be considered when the young person is too ill or impaired to communicate them. NICE16 also recommends the use of advanced care plans (ACP) for all young people with life limited conditions. An ACP can be used not just to record a young person's wishes and preferences, but also to document how he or she communicates. A second recommendation is therefore that all young people with long-term health conditions should have an ACP. However, this comes with a caveat: just as with the law and guidance mentioned, ACPs are only beneficial if health professionals firstly understand their purpose and secondly use them. A concern repeatedly raised to me by paediatricians is that some paediatricians wrongly assume that an ACP always means a young person should not have active healthcare, just palliative care. This is a wrong assumption. Adam's experience is also relevant. When he moved from one health region to another, his detailed ACP, written and updated regularly over many years by his old health team with Adam's full participation, was ignored by his new healthcare team because it came from a different NHS region. Adam's wishes and preferences were consequently ignored when he became critically ill, as was important information about his ability to communicate and participate in decisions. Safeguards are needed to protect young people in this situation.

For all its failings a statutory equivalent to the MCA for young people under 16 could be the answer, placing statutory duties on paediatricians and other professionals to facilitate young people's participation in decisions (House of Lords, 2014b). To avoid the failings of the MCA a substantive and probably compulsory programme of education and training for all professionals working with young people would be needed.

As Adam's life and death showed, and as senior paediatricians from around the UK in my research confirmed, fulfilling young people's rights to participate in decisions about their healthcare is not just a legal obligation, it is a matter of life and death. Proper education and training of health professionals in young people's participation rights is essential, as is compassionate and wide-ranging communication by health professionals.

Notes
[1]   A national regional or hospital providing specialist care.

2   A local hospital providing generalist care.

3   Article 12, United Nations (1989) Convention on the Rights of the Child.

4   'State Parties shall assure to the child who is capable of forming his or her views the right to express those views freely in all matters affecting the child, the views of the child being given due weight in accordance with the age and maturity of the child'. Article 12, United Nations (1989) Convention on the Rights of the Child.

5   Ratification is the formal process whereby a state becomes legally bound by international law.

6   The UK signed the UNCRC on 19th April 1990 and ratified on 16th December 1991.

7   The Scottish Government announced in its Programme of Government published on 4th September 2018 that the UNCRC would be incorporated into Scots Law, www.gov.scot/publications/delivering-today-investing-tomorrow-governments-programme-scotland-2018-19/ [Last accessed: 26th January 2019].

8   International treaties can be incorporated into domestic law in the UK through an Act of Parliament.

9   See for example, Section 1, Children and Young People (Scotland) Act 2014 and The Children Act 1989.

10 Reporting should happen every five years, but there is a backlog.

11 Article 44, United Nations (1989) Convention on the Rights of the Child.

12 In the UK, a government report and a civil society report is prepared for each of the four nation states and then combined into a single UK report.

13 Office for the High Commissioner United Nations Human Rights, https://www.ohchr.org/EN/HRBodies/CRC/Pages/CRCIndex.aspx [Last accessed: 21st May 2020].

14 UN, 2009: CRC/C/CGC/12, para 15.

15 UN, 2015: CRC/C/GBR/5, para 44.

16 UN, 2009: CRC/C/CGC/12, para 15.

17 UN, 2009: CRC/C/CGC/12, para 15.

18 UN, 2009: CRC/C/CGC/12, para 28.

19 UN, 2009: CRC/C/CGC/12, para 98.

20 UN, 2009: CRC/C/CGC/12, para 16.

21 In Scotland the relevant legislation is the Adults with Incapacity (Scotland) Act 2000.

22 HM Gov, Mental Capacity Act Code of Practice (2016).

23 Section 1, Mental Capacity Act 2005.

24 Section 1(3) Mental Capacity Act 2005.

25 In Scotland the relevant legislation is the Age of Legal Capacity (Scotland) Act 1991.

26 Gillick v West Norfolk and Wisebech Area Health Authority [1985] 3 All ER 402.

27 The GMC has a statutory duty to regulate the training and practice of all UK medical doctors under the Medical Act 1983 c 54.

28 GMC, Professionalism in action, Good Medical Practice, para 5, www.gmc-uk.org/ethical-guidance/ethical-guidance-for-doctors/good-medical-practice/professionalism-in-action [Last accessed: 26th January 2019]

29 GMC, Professionalism in action, Good Medical Practice, para 14.

30 GMC, Professionalism in action, Good Medical Practice, para 14.

31 Medical royal colleges oversee the training and education of health professionals within a particular speciality.

32 The National Institute for Health and Care Excellence is a Non Departmental Public Body tasked with providing national guidance and advice to improve health and social care.

33 'The professionals' first duty is to respect life and the health of patients by preserving life, restoring health and preventing disease'. Larcher, V., Craig, F., Bhogal, K., Wilkinson, D. and Brierley, J. (2015) Making decisions to limit treatment in life-limiting and life-threatening conditions in children: A framework for practice. *Archives of Disease in Childhood*, 100, s1-23 para 2.4.1.

34 A fully qualified doctor with significant experience in their speciality.

35 An experienced 'junior doctor' who will soon complete their training and be eligible to become a consultant.

36 For example, the Paediatric Intensive Care Society; the British Paediatric Respiratory Society and British Paediatric Neurology Association.

37 Specialists in conditions affecting the brain and nervous system.

38 Specialists in the treatment of children and young people generally.

39 Specialists in conditions affecting lungs.

40 Specialists in the treatment of illnesses related to the endocrine system.

41 Specialists in the treatment of patients where the chemical processes in the body do not work correctly.

42 Specialist in the treatment of children with cancer.

43 A paediatrician working in accident and emergency.

44 A paediatrician working with children and young people with life limiting conditions.

45 A paediatrician specialising in the care of newborn infants under the age of one month.

46 The GMC register of doctors eligible for appointment as a consultant. See www.gmc-uk.org/doctors/register/information_on_the_specialist_register.asp [Last accessed: 12th June 2017].

47 s.6 Equality Act, 2010, c.15.

48 'Islands of development' is a term used by doctors to describe when a child with a neurological impairment develops has abilities in one area but has impairment in another.

49 A heuristic as a rule derived often from experience of similar cases used to simplify decision-making.

50 *Adam Talking About Rights* (2010) film produced for the Scottish Alliance for Children's Rights.

References

Cuttini, M., Nadai, M., Kaminski, M., Hansen, G., de Leeuw, R., Lenoir, S., Persson, J., Rebagliato, M., Reid, M., de Vonderweid, U., Lenard, H.G., Orzalesi, M.D. and Saracci, R. (2000) End-of-life decisions in neonatal intensive care: Physicians' self-reported practices in seven European countries. *The Lancet*, 355 (9221), pp 2112–8.

DWP (2012) *Family resources survey United Kingdom 2010/2011*. London: Department for Work and Pensions, p 79.

GMC (2011) *The state of medical education and practice in the UK*. London: GMC, p 21.

GMC (2018) *0–18 years: Guidance for all doctors*. London: GMC. Available from: www.gmc-uk.org/ethical-guidance/ethical-guidance-for-doctors/0–18-years, para 3 [Last accessed: 30th January 2019].

House of Lords (2014a) Select Committee on Mental Capacity Act 2005, Report of Session 2013–14, Mental Capacity Act 2005: Post-legislative scrutiny.

House of Lords (2014b) *Mental Capacity Act 2005: Post-legislative scrutiny*. Select Committee on the Mental Capacity Act 2005, Report of Session 2013–14, HL Paper 139 Available from: https://publications.parliament.uk/pa/ld201314/ldselect/ldmentalcap/139/139.pdf [Last accessed: 30th January 2019].

Kline, R. (2014) *The 'snowy white peaks' of the NHS: A survey of the discrimination in governance and leadership and the potential impact on patient care in London and England*. London: Middlesex University.

Larcher, V., Craig, F., Bhogal, K., Wilkinson, D. and Brierley, J. (2015) Making decisions to limit treatment in life-limiting and life-threatening conditions in children: A framework for practice. *Archives of Disease in Childhood*, 100, s1-23

Mebane, E.W., Oman, R.F., Kroonen, L.T. and Goldstein, M.K. (1999) The influence of physician race, age, and gender on physician attitudes toward advance care directives and preferences for end-of-life decision-making. *Journal of the American Geriatrics Society*, 47 (5), pp 579–91.

NICE (2016) *End of life care for infants, children and young people with life-limiting conditions: Planning and management*, NG61.

Picton-Howell, Z. (2018) *UK paediatricians' medical decision-making for severely disabled children – A socio-legal study*. PhD thesis, School of Law, University of Edinburgh.

Priest, N., Esmail, A., Williams, D.R., Norman, F.S. and Norman, L.S. (2015) Promoting equality for ethnic minority NHS staff – What works? *BMJ*, 351, h3297.

RCPCH (2004) *Withholding life sustaining treatment in children, A framework for practice*. 2nd edition. London: Royal College of Paediatrics and Child Health.

RCPCH (2013) *RCPCH medical workforce census for 2011*. London: Royal College of Paediatrics and Child Health, p 46.

RCPCH (2014) *RCPCH medical workforce census 2013*. London: Royal College of Paediatrics and Child Health, Main Findings, p 2.

UN (United Nations) (2009) Committee on the Rights of the Child, *General Comment No. 12, the right of the child to be heard*. CRC/C/CGC/12, para 15.

UN (2015) Committee on the Rights of the Child, *Consideration of reports submitted by States parties under article 44 due in 2014 United Kingdom*, CRC/C/GBR/5, para 44

Wilkinson, D. and Truog, R.D. (2013) The luck of the draw: Physician-related variability in end-of-life decision-making in intensive care. *Intensive Care Medicine*, 39 (6), 1128–32, at p 1129.

PART II

Participation in national projects and programmes

3

'Giving young people a voice': lessons from the NHS England Youth Forum

Lisa Whiting, Sheila Roberts,
Kath Evans and Julia Petty

Introduction

Young people want to be involved in the decisions that impact on them and their health service provision (Royal College of Paediatrics and Child Health [RCPCH], 2017) – a youth forum is one way of enabling this. This chapter will initially focus on the background and development of youth forums/councils; secondly, an overview of the National Health Service England Youth Forum (NHSEYF) will be provided with the perspectives of Kath Evans (Experience of Care Lead, NHS England[1] (NHSE) – Maternity, Infants, Children and Young People) and NHSEYF members being integrated. Thirdly, an evaluative mixed methods study (undertaken by the University of Hertfordshire (UH)) will be briefly presented. Finally, the chapter will present the Youth Forum Wheel (YFW) that was developed as a direct result of the research; the YFW is offered to health professionals and young people who may be implementing and/or managing youth forums. It aims to provide insight into the underpinning components of success, each of these will be discussed and their practical application considered.

The development of youth forums

A youth forum has been described as being in existence to:

> represent the views of young people, giving young people the opportunity to have a voice, discuss issues, engage with decision makers and contribute to improving and developing services for young people. (NHS England, 2015a, p 5)

One of the longest running youth forums that is widely recognised within the UK is the Northern Ireland Youth Forum which was established in 1979 by the Department of Education; this organisation has continued to develop and has a very active membership (Northern Ireland Youth Forum, 2019). In 1999, a youth forum was held in The Hague to enable 132 young people, representing 111 countries, to offer their thoughts and opinions on a range of key organisations (including the United Nations, as well as governmental and non-governmental bodies) about areas such as health, human rights and education (Youth Forum, 1999). In the same year, UNESCO introduced their first youth forum event – this has since been held every two years at the headquarters in Paris; it is open to all young people and aims to provide:

> an innovative, ongoing opportunity for youth to work in dialogue with UNESCO, to shape and direct the Organization's approach and to present their concerns and ideas to Member States. (UNESCO, 2019)[2]

While there has been some interchangeable usage of the terms 'youth forum' and 'youth council', the latter is normally linked with governmental bodies (Collins et al, 2016). Matthews (2001) provides a historical development of youth councils within the UK – a summary is provided in Box 3.1.

Box 3.1: The development of youth councils within the UK

1940s–1950s: The establishment of youth parliaments throughout the UK; in 1949, 240 youth councils were in existence.

1980s: Following The Thompson Report (Department of Education and Science, 1982), another surge of youth council establishment occurred; however, many were not underpinned by robust structures, so did not last for more than a few years.

1990s: Youth councils began to develop more strongly in the 1990s; for example, in 1996, the National Youth Agency started to provide, on request, information about youth forums (Matthews and Limb, 1998). The growth within England and Wales was rather disorganised, whereas Scotland adopted a more structured approach.

(Prime source: Matthews, 2001)

There are a range of established models aimed at facilitating children and young people's participation; for example, Hart (1992) offered a 'ladder' designed to encourage those working with children and young people to think more closely about the nature and purpose of their participation in community activities. The ladder depicts eight levels that outline different forms and stages ('manipulation'; 'decoration'; 'tokenism'; 'assigned but informed'; consulted and informed'; 'adult initiated, shared decisions with children'; 'child-initiated and directed'; 'child-initiated, shared decisions with adults') – the first three steps relate to non-participation whereas the higher rungs refer to 'real' participation. In contrast, the Children's Commissioner (Office of the Children's Commissioner, 2015) developed a Wheel of Participation to recognise children and young people's participation through the stages of inform, consult or involve. The different models, wheels or ladders, are further discussed by Aspland (2015). In terms of youth councils/ forums, it has been suggested that there are six different types that enable youth participation (Box 3.2); this contribution is of particular value as work in this area is so limited.

Box 3.2: Types of youth councils/forums

Feeder or constituent organisations:
Focuses on engaging young people in a range of decision-making that falls within the remit of the local authority.

Shadow organisations:
Run alongside a committee/organisation that is adult-based and would include, for example, a local youth parliament.

Issue-specific organisations:
Established by a specific organisation with the aim of involving young people in decisions that are central to it. This is the approach that would be most closely aligned to health focussed youth forums.

Community-development organisations:
Focuses on local issues that are of concern to young people.

Group-specific organisations:
Involves young people who all have a specific issue/concern in common – for example, those with disabilities or those who are lesbian, gay or bisexual.

Young-people initiated organisations:
Developed, organised and coordinated by young people; this model is less frequently used.

(Matthews and Limb, 1998)

Since 1979, the number of youth forums has grown considerably within the UK; it is estimated that there are now more than 620 youth councils/forums, covering areas such as local government, boroughs and county councils (NHS England, 2015a); the ages of the young people involved (whether the forums are related to health or other societal issues) are normally between 11 and 25 years of age.

Background: NHS England Youth Forum

In order to meet the national agenda of ensuring young people are represented, involved and have their voice heard across the whole of NHS England, the NHSEYF was established in 2013. Discussions initially took place with key stakeholders from NHS England (Patient Experience and Public and Patient Voice), Public Health England[3] and the Department of Health[4] – a tripartite approach being adopted to avoid repetition across the different organisations. The NHSEYF aimed to meet key objectives of involving young people but also to act as a role model for other organisations such as Clinical Commissioning Groups.[5]

The British Youth Council (BYC), who has national coverage and an outreach of approximately seven million young people, was given the responsibility of the day-to-day management of the NHSEYF. The BYC works closely with a range of other youth sector partners, for example Whizz-Kidz, National Children's Bureau, Brook, Sense and the Council for Disabled Children – representatives from these organisations formed an Adult Reference Group. The Adult Reference Group, which was convened prior to the recruitment of the NHSEYF young people, initially met every six to eight weeks to act in an advisory capacity to facilitate the establishment of the NHSEYF. The Adult Reference Group has since been dissolved as its role is complete; however, the NHSEYF continues to be supported by the patient and public voice team internally at NHS England.

The purpose of the NHS England Youth Forum is to:

- work with a diverse range of young people who can bring their perspectives and experiences of healthcare services;
- seek advice from young people about key areas of strategic healthcare policies and national programmes;
- enable young people to hold commissioners and executive board members to account;
- listen to young people's experiences and ideas for health service improvement;

- work with children and young people and their respective communities to understand how better services can be commissioned.

The NHSEYF initially comprised of 20 young people, aged 15–21; this has since increased to 25 (aged 14–23) in order to enable good and consistent attendance at the residential weekends, but to also give the young people a degree of flexibility in terms of their study commitments. BYC was responsible for recruiting the initial members; nine young people were elected by the BYC from the nine English regions, each of these young people already held roles as, for example, youth councillors, young mayors or members of the UK Youth Parliament. They demonstrated that they were confident communicators and able to effectively challenge issues. The remaining 11 places were appointed based on the strength of the young person's application, but also ensuring that there was fair geographical, gender, age and disability representation across England; applications were received from approximately 200 interested young people and the final 11 members were selected by the original nine young people who had been appointed by BYC.

The NHSEYF young people communicate with each other through pre-arranged residential meetings held three times a year as well as via a 'closed' Facebook page (supported and monitored by a BYC employee) and the *Wednesday Weekly* email (a form of newsletter); in order to reach out to a wider population of children and young people, there is also an 'open' Facebook page.[6] Outside of the pre-arranged residential events, the young people are invited to a variety of meetings and conferences where they are able to engage with key stakeholders across a range of healthcare services. For further details about the NHSEYF please refer to their website.[7]

Since its inception, the NHSEYF has played a key role in facilitating the implementation of locally based youth forums via events such as 'The Big Youth Forum Meet Up'[8] and their *Cooking up a Youth Forum* film.[9] Table 3.1 provides examples of locally based youth forms that have been established within NHS England Trusts, and Table 3.2 details the type of work that has been undertaken.

Table 3.1: Examples of youth forums based in NHS Trusts within England

Youth forum	Age range	Aims
Harrogate and District NHS Foundation Trust: https://www.hdft.nhs.uk/about/education-liaison/youth-forum/	13–19	To make services welcoming to children and young people. To enable young people to understand their healthcare rights. To make healthcare services more accessible for young people.
Chelsea and Westminster NHS Foundation Trust: https://www.chelwest.nhs.uk/services/childrens-services/youth-forum-meeting	11–18	To provide a safe and confidential forum space for young patients aged 11–18 years to come together and express their views and opinions about their hospital experience and work together to help improve services.
Great Ormond Street Hospital for Children NHS Foundation Trust: https://www.gosh.nhs.uk/teenagers/teengosh-community/young-peoples-forum	10–21	To consider what the hospital should be taking action on, what they are doing well and get updates on how views and opinions have impacted on care and services.

Table 3.2: Example of the work of a local youth forum based in an NHS England Trust

Youth forum	Activities
Blackpool's Victoria's voice	This local forum is run by a youth worker; the members (aged 11–16) meet on a monthly basis and have all been a patient at the Blackpool Victoria Hospital; the focus of the forum is the enhancement of the hospital and community services. One scheme that was undertaken was the involvement of young people in the teaching and induction of doctors; the young people developed a 'Top Tips' (Blackpool Teaching Hospitals NHS Foundation Trust, 2018) card that focused on key areas to consider when communicating with children and young people. The forum members gave a presentation and provided copies of the card to the doctors. While the project was not without its initial challenges, the motivation and commitment of the young people, as well as the forum facilitators, meant that the initiative was met with success and received positive feedback. In addition, the forum has been involved in a wide range of other initiatives that have included the selection and recruitment of consultant paediatricians and ward managers as well as work with a local special needs school to enhance disability awareness with health staff (this work was recognised by the Department of Education).

Outside of the UK, countries such as Australia are working hard to ensure that the voice of the young person is heard – for example, in September 2018, Consumers Health Forum of Australia (CHF) held their inaugural Youth Health Forum which brought together young people aged 16–30 to share their views on the Australian health and social care system (CHF, 2018).

A NHSEYF facilitator's perspective

In this section, Kath Evans (Experience of Care Lead, NHS England (NHSE) – Maternity, Infants, Children and Young People) provides a unique perspective on the NHSEYF. Three key areas are addressed: recruitment, impact and challenges.

Recruitment

The young people are recruited to the NHSEYF with the help of the BYC which has the capacity to reach a wider cohort of young people through social media, such as Facebook and Twitter, rather than being reliant on more traditional advertising methods such as the NHS England newsletters. From the beginning, young people (the nine who had been elected by the BYC, from the nine English regions), were involved in reviewing applications from other young people. The application form is kept simple to ensure that it is accessible and inclusive. The young people are instrumental in identifying people that they think have significant contributions to make to the health agenda. Young people are initially recruited for one year, and they can then choose to continue for a second year; after the second year they become an alumni member. It is essential that connections are maintained but fresh voices are recruited to the youth forum.

Between 2014 and 2017 the NHSEYF membership represented a cross section of society with minority groups often over-represented compared to the wider population (BYC and NHS England, 2017). Demographics are summarised in Tables 3.3, 3.4. 3.5 and 3.6.

Table 3.3: Ethnicity of NHSEYF members

Ethnicity	Percentage/number
White British	64.3%, n=45
Asian	10%, n=7
Black African	7%, n=5
Others, for example other white/mixed race/ Middle Eastern	14.3%, n=10
Prefer not to say	4.3%, n=3

Table 3.4: Age of NHSEYF members

Age	Percentage/number	Age	Percentage/number
14	4.3%, n=3	20	4.3%, n=3
15	8.6%, n=6	21	5.7%, n=4
16	22.9%, n=16	22	4.3%, n=3
17	22.9%, n=16	23	4.3%, n=3
18	14.3%, n=10	24	5.7%, n=4
19	11.4%, n=8	25	1.4%, n=1

Table 3.5: Geographical location of NHSEYF members

Geographical location	Percentage/number
North East	4.3%, n=3
North West	17%, n=12
Yorkshire and Humberside	10%, n=7
West Midlands	14.3%, n=10
East Midlands	8.6%, n=6
East of England	2.8%, n=2
South West	20%, n=14
London	14.3%, n=10
South East	8.6%, n=6

Table 3.6: Disability of NHSEYF members

Disability	Percentage/number
Yes	72.8%, n=51
No	21.4%, n=15
Prefer not to say	5.7%, n=4

Working with the BYC has enabled the recruitment of a diverse range of young people, including those who have faced substantive life difficulties such as mental health challenges, physical problems, caring responsibilities as well as those who are considered more vulnerable and 'hard to reach'. One member of the NHSEYF was once heard to say, "I'm not hard to reach, Kath. You can get a bus to my housing estate, it's just that you choose not to get that bus to my housing estate." This emphasises the need to use a breadth of approaches to enable the participation of young people.

Impact

The BYC, along with key personnel from NHS England, has been instrumental in ensuring that the voices of young people are truly and accurately heard. A booklet and posters reflecting youth rights in healthcare (NHS England, 2016) have been widely distributed to professionals across England. The ongoing collaborative relationship between young people and healthcare professionals has helped to move health agendas forward. Moreover, there is evidence that young people's contribution is not only valued, but that their work is having an impact on the health service agenda; for example:

2014
- A change was made to the NHS complaints policy, ensuring that it is now clear that young people can make complaints in their own right and need to be taken seriously.[10]
- A series of posters were produced outlining young people's rights in healthcare.[11]

2014–15
- A social campaign run by the NHSEYF called 'Dear NHS' was created. It enabled young people across the country to talk about their healthcare services (for example[12]).
- The development of a short document to enable young people to challenge commissioners about the transition to adult services.[13]

- A drive to advocate for better mental health services for young people.

2015–16
- The development of resources for commissioners to help them involve young people in strategic decision-making.
- Work was undertaken to refresh the 'You're Welcome' assurance standards for children and young people's health services.[14]

2016–17
- Resources were produced to support general practice (GP) and primary care to involve young people in improving healthcare services.
- A one-page good practice guide to underpin high-quality care was developed, and sent to all of the Vanguard programmes within the NHS.[15]
- A campaign, encouraging young people to think about their own wellbeing (#yourhealthinyourhands), was instigated.

More recently, the NHSEYF has been involved in challenging the barriers to young people volunteering within the NHS; for example, the work with the #iwill campaign[16] is inspiring NHS organisations to facilitate volunteering roles for young people. The NHSEYF members have shared their perspective on youth volunteering and have advocated for youth voice, community engagement and peer support in relation to volunteering opportunities.

The NHSEYF are acting as ambassadors; lines of enquiry or 'killer' questions have been developed that encourage organisations to challenge themselves and develop youth volunteering. For example, Birmingham Women's and Children's NHS Foundation Trust are now liaising with local groups to enable young people to volunteer.[17] Sheffield's sexual health service[18] enables some health education to be carried out by peers rather than healthcare professionals who could be 20 or 30 years older than the young people seeking advice.

The NHSEYF is currently involved in championing the voice of the child and young person in safeguarding processes. One of the benefits of the youth forum is that the health experts build a relationship with the young people; an example is the use of residential weekends to help facilitate this. The health experts may be zip wiring with the young people one moment and asking their opinions the next, and this all helps to build a trusting relationship. Many of the NHSEYF members have used safeguarding processes, and through this they have come into contact with healthcare professionals, the police and with social work; however, nobody normally asks the young people, 'How was the process?' By involving the NHSEYF members, a greater understanding is established. Whereas healthcare professionals may focus on the more concerning aspects of safeguarding, sexual exploitation or being a vulnerable child, the young people raised different challenges, for example, bullying was an important issue for them. The NHSEYF are continuing to work alongside NHS England to challenge and hold them to account as new safeguarding reforms are embedded across the healthcare system. This is another example of the NHSEYF working alongside more professionally led and driven steering groups and programmes of work.

Challenges

One of the significant aspects of working with young people in a health context is the use of language. Young people talk of health and wellbeing in very broad terms and do not necessarily understand the differences between the roles and responsibilities of organisations such as NHS England, Public Health England, Department of Health and Social Care, Health Education England[19] or the Care Quality Commission[20] – nor should there be an expectation that they do. It is NHS England's responsibility to ensure that the right connections are made, that the young people's issues are taken to the relevant organisations and that invitations to appropriate events are provided; in order to have a positive impact on healthcare services, these connections need to work well – at executive level there is a requirement and responsibility to engage with, and listen to, the public (NHS England, 2015b). When the NHSEYF attended Westminster Abbey for the NHS's 70th birthday, Simon Stevens,

Chief Executive of NHS England, was asked to greet the young people – this was very much appreciated.

Another challenge for the members of the NHSEYF relates to geography. The young people are supported and encouraged to work on national campaigns; however, when they return home, they may receive a mixed response. Young people may, for example, contact their local GP or NHS Trust, and while some may be made to feel very welcome, others may not. It is therefore important to provide ongoing support and build on success – for example, one NHSEYF member is working with a patient and public participation group in her GP surgery; another is working with his local NHS Trust hospital to set up their own youth forum.

NHSEYF members' perspective

To further illustrate the experiences of being involved in the NHSEYF, narratives from three young people (Dominic, Amy, Ethan) are presented (Boxes 3.3, 3.4 and 3.5).

Box 3.3: The voice of Dominic

Hello, my name is Dominic. I'm 23, I work at Student Minds and I am a member of the NHS England Youth Forum.

I got involved with the NHSEYF because I love the NHS. I believe in patient-centred, compassionate healthcare that is free and accessible. I've benefitted from a range of NHS services – GPs, specialist care and sexual health – and have had really positive experiences, particularly with the latter. But that doesn't mean the NHS couldn't be even better.

I wanted to be involved with the NHSEYF to improve how the NHS provides services to LGBTQ+ individuals, students and young people as well as to shape how it links up with Higher Education Institutions.

Because of being in the NHS Youth Forum I have been afforded a plethora of opportunities to shape the work the NHS does. I have spoken at an All-Party Parliamentary Group on 'managing long-term conditions at university', highlighting the challenges and experiences of students, the barriers they face in accessing help and support and outlining the current student mental health landscape. I attended NHS Expo [Health and Care Innovation Expo;[21] www.england.nhs.uk/expo/about/], the annual convention of the NHS – where I met and spoke to a range of professionals in the NHS about the work they do and how they can better engage with young people. I attended the NHS Annual General Meeting and asked Sir Malcolm Grant, the then Chairman of the NHS, about how they are planning to improve Gender Identity Clinics and the care offered to trans people. I consulted on the NHS Long Term Plan, the priorities of the NHS and how it can and should embed youth engagement across its services. I was afforded these opportunities and many more because I chose to get involved in the work of the NHSEYF.

Box 3.4: The voice of Amy

In 2014, I did something spontaneous; I applied to be a member in the inaugural year of the NHSEYF. For a girl who hadn't previously used public transport, was unconfident in group environments and struggled to verbally assert her views, it was a bold and brave move. Being a member of the NHSEYF shaped my life; when I began, I was feeling isolated with rock-bottom self-esteem, but I left in 2016 transformed, with a reignited love for learning, life-long friends and a sense of feeling 'valued'. I hadn't anticipated my personal progression – all I had wanted was to improve healthcare experiences for children and young people. Nor did I anticipate the wider level of change that we [NHSEYF] could have at a national level. It amazed me to see that so many other like-minded young people both in the NHSEYF and other networks strived to spread the participation message. It was, and remains, astounding to see those services, who truly embrace the value of participation of young people, develop to create better care and experiences for the service, staff, volunteers and patients.

Participating in the NHSEYF gave me an opportunity to network and gain understanding of the variety of roles that NHS England offers. It acted as a catalyst, enabling me to develop further engagement and roles in numerous organisations. The foundations built from NHSEYF supported me to pursue my dreams; I am now a trainee Psychological Wellbeing Practitioner in conjunction to studying an MSci Applied Psychology (Clinical) at University. I love my new roles and am excited for the future. I still commit my spare time to volunteering as those roles continue to hold a special place in my heart.

Box 3.5: The voice of Ethan

Hello, my name is Ethan. I am 24 and I live in London and am originally from Birmingham.

I have lived with dyslexia and have been on the autistic spectrum all of my life. This has meant learning that the health system is not always going to work for you, unless you engage with it, challenge it and try to make it better, not just for myself but primarily for young people who come after me.

In 2017 when I was six months into remission from testicular cancer, I decided that the experience I had, and was having, needed to be changed and challenged. I was thankful to have an amazing charity, CLIC Sargent, there to support me and provide a platform for me to participate. CLIC Sargent also encouraged me to apply to the NHSEYF in June 2017. In September 2017 I also joined the civil service.

So, you might ask why I work in a full-time job and volunteer, give up my weekends for long days in random parts of the country. I could answer that in a few ways. When you are 23 years old and an opportunity comes up which is only for people up to 25 years wouldn't you give it a shot? Cancer has made me appreciate that my life can be taken away from me either permanently or to such an extent that when I return, the world will have moved on, doors may no longer be open. So, give it a shot, I hopefully have made a decent contribution over the years sharing my experience.

Evaluating young peoples' views of the NHSEYF

This section will provide an overview of a research study that was undertaken by the UH between July 2015 and September 2016. The study sought to ascertain the views and experiences of young people in relation to being members of the NHSEYF and the strategies used to influence health service provision (please refer to Whiting et al, 2018 for a full overview of the research). From this study emerged the YFW that provides a model, detailing components of success and their practical application.

A mixed method evaluative approach, utilising quantitative and qualitative data collection approaches, enabled different perspectives to be appreciated (Moule and Goodman, 2014). Quantitative data collection was undertaken via the development and distribution of Activity Logs (Appendix 3.1) that were to be completed over a three-month period; all 25 NHSEYF members were sent the logs, with nine young people completing and returning them. The logs allowed documentation of the activities (time spent on them, as well as the location and cost). All 25 NHSEYF members were also invited to participate in a face-to-face semi-structured interview to further facilitate the exploration of their experiences; eight young people agreed; one person completed both the Activity Logs as well as an interview. Ethical approval was granted by the UH (protocol numbers: HSK/SF/UH/00119; HSK/SF/UH/02383).

Descriptive statistics were used to analyse the quantitative data from the Activity Logs. The six-stage 'bottom-up' Qualitative Process of Data Analysis (Creswell, 2012) was applied to analyse the interview transcripts as it is clearly structured and is suited to an evaluative approach. Seven themes emerged from the data and these were used to inform the development of the YFW.

The Youth Forum Wheel (Whiting et al, 2016a)

The YFW (Figure 3.1) depicts the seven 'components of success' – these were identified by the young people themselves (via the data collection and analysis processes) as being central to the success of a youth forum. The representation has a circular structure to illustrate the equal value and connectivity that each

Figure 3.1: The Youth Forum Wheel

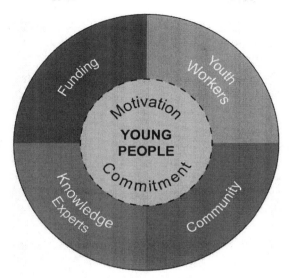

The Youth Forum Wheel (YFW)

Source: Whiting et al (2016a)

component has. Firstly, the young people themselves are of fundamental importance; in order to acknowledge this they are placed at the core of the YFW. Two of the other components of success are qualities that the young people possess ('motivation' and 'commitment'). The other four are external factors that are integral to the Youth Forum achievements ('community'; 'funding'; 'knowledge experts' and 'youth workers'); the relevance and application of all of these seven areas are discussed in the next section.

Application of the YFW

Young people

The selection and recruitment of forum members is important and requires clear criteria to ensure that the young people understand the commitment and motivation that may be required; the participation of young people in the recruitment processes undoubtedly strengthens them, helping to ensure that young people are working together to meet a common aim. In addition, it is important to achieve appropriate representation in terms of gender, culture and geographical location – this is something that can be lacking (Matthews, 2001).

As is the case with many other youth forums, the NHSEYF members gave their time freely, willingly and with enthusiasm, without wanting any financial remuneration. Most of them had previously been involved in other local volunteer initiatives (some of which were health-related) – this had, in many instances, led directly to the application for NHSEYF membership. This had two consequences; firstly, it meant that the participants had some prior insight into the expectations of a volunteer role, and this may have, in turn, contributed to their understanding of the need for commitment and motivation. Secondly, it facilitated a bi-directional dissemination of the NHSEYF work so that national initiatives could be implemented at a local level and vice versa. For example, the previously mentioned booklet and posters reflecting young people's rights in healthcare (NHS England, 2016) have been widely distributed across England; in another instance, an NHSEYF member had been involved, in her local area, with the making of a film relating to mental health awareness – this had been shown to her peers at one of the NHSEYF residential weekends and it had inspired others to think about mental health wellbeing in the context of their own locality.

Motivation

Young people's motivation to be involved in volunteering is based on: personal satisfaction, collective efficacy and contributing to shared national values (Sherrod et al, 2002); this was certainly the case with the NHSEYF. Their participation had meant that there had been personal growth and development as well as the achievement of shared local and national objectives. While there are many reasons why a young person may wish to join a youth forum (for example, it could stem from personal healthcare experiences or it could be to facilitate future career aspirations), motivation must also come from the absolute belief in the importance of enabling the voices of young people to be heard.

Commitment

This aspect of the YFW concurs with findings from previous research – Salusky et al (2014) found that at some point the majority of young people experienced challenges in terms of their volunteering commitment and could waiver in their responsibilities. However, the NHSEYF members' commitment was strong, ongoing and was also, in many instances, extended to other organisations; one participant commented, "You can't just say, 'Oh, actually I'm busy.'"

The young people spoke about the length of their term of office and it was generally agreed that being a member for a two-year period was advantageous as this enabled them to not only gain insight, knowledge and familiarity with NHS England, but it also offered more opportunities to participate in activities; they felt that this was important as if they were, for example, in school Years 11 or 13 when their personal time may be needed to focus on their examinations, a second year of office gave more scope for involvement.

Community

Key findings from previous studies (Matthews, 2001; Collins et al, 2016) revealed that the needs of local communities were being met via the work of youth councils. A significant aspect of the NHSEYF work related to the 'ripple effect' (something that was described by a previous NHS England Youth Forum member in an earlier research study, Whiting et al, 2016b); in other words collaborating with others at both a local and national level so that the youth forum work was disseminated. All of the young people had a good knowledge and awareness of their local area that had come from growing up in their community. They had gained knowledge of the physical geography but had also developed friendships with peers as well as relationships with key people, the latter sometimes being as a result of accessing health services or being involved in local initiatives. This community knowledge should not be underestimated in terms of a youth forum maximising its potential and fulfilling local needs. One participant in our work gave the example of how his knowledge of his local environment had helped him to engage with a GP surgery to raise awareness of health issues to young people (in particular mental health and teenage cancer). Another aspect was the community spirit that the forum generated; the participants vocalised how they worked together with a common aim and how they had formed some very strong friendships.

Funding

Finances are inevitably required to underpin the running of a youth forum; this may not just include the cost of venue hire, refreshments, travel, but can also mean that there are expenses associated with the implementation of initiatives as well as staff time. A youth forum needs to carefully consider its role and aim within the context of the available financial support to ensure that the goals are achievable and realistic. The NHSEYF young people had their personal expenses covered but there was no expectation, or desire, from any participant to be paid for their time.

Knowledge experts

It has been suggested that the role of the adult should be that of facilitator or mediator, working alongside young people in a supportive role (Wyness, 2009). The need for adult support to enable young people's opinions to be heard and acted on has been recognised (NHS England, 2015a); this suggests that one of the key roles of the adult involved in youth forums is to build bridges between young people and those in authority in order to bring about change.

In terms of the NHSEYF, the knowledge experts were NHS England employees who had tremendous insight into the structure and processes of the NHS – without this vital 'interpretation', young people may not gain the necessary insight into the NHS quite so quickly and, therefore, outcomes may take longer to achieve.

The NHSEYF members mentioned their presence at the residential weekends, giving examples of how they had facilitated group work or decision-making – the latter particularly relating to the focus of the NHSEYF work. In addition, the NHS employees had a presence with the young people at conferences and other key activities across the country.

Youth workers

The young people all spoke of the support and guidance provided by the BYC youth workers. Their role differed to that of the knowledge experts in that they led the day-to-day management of the NHSEYF, communication with the young people being a key aspect – this was via a variety of strategies, including discussions at the residential weekends, personal emails and telephone calls. However, the prime route was via the 'closed' Facebook page and the *Wednesday Weekly* email; these mechanisms were mainly used to pass on information and also to ask the young people for their opinions and comments on key documents. There was evidence that the participants liked this form of communication and responded well to it.

The youth workers also arranged many of the NHSEYF's activities as well as associated travel; the ongoing contact that the members had with the youth workers meant that a rapport was established and that the young people felt comfortable, secure and able to voice any queries or concerns.

Conclusions

The NHSEYF offers a unique model and is ideally placed to share examples of good practice (both within the UK and further afield). These include: healthcare professionals developing trusting relationships with young people to facilitate the vocalisation of youth voice; the utilisation of mechanisms such as social media to convey key messages; being creative with short films and narratives so that they are engaging and points are appropriately conveyed; young people and healthcare professionals truly working together to enhance healthcare services. The NHSEYF has offered a secure base for role-modelling how to facilitate the participation of young people. It is not without its challenges and therefore more youth organisations need to work alongside NHS England to ensure that *everyone* knows that engaging with young people is possible and is achievable.

Young people account for approximately one fifth of the UK population (Office of National Statistics, 2017); as health services continue to evolve, it is essential that they continue to have their voice heard, at both an individual and strategic level. Some areas of healthcare already have good levels of engagement with young people, but, unfortunately, this is not yet consistent. It can be difficult, for example, for young people to be heard within health settings that are outside of a large hospital environment – it is clear that young people need the appropriate support to enable them to develop their skills and to be able to voice their views. The YFW is offered as a framework that has the potential to inform others and to enable the voice of young people to be heard; by considering the components of success, thought can be given to the key areas required to underpin a youth forum. The financial backing and adult expertise should not be underestimated; without this, young people are less likely to be able to access the resources, training and support that are required to enable them to confidently assume their membership role.

The NHSEYF has developed rapidly and successfully – this is undoubtedly due to the total commitment, motivation and enthusiasm of all those involved, especially the young people who have given their time so willingly. Most importantly, the work of the NHSEYF has ensured that the voices of young people are now being more widely listened to:

> 'I think the key point is showing adults that young people want to have their voices heard.' (Matt)

Acknowledgements

The authors are very grateful to the young people who participated in the research. Thank you.

Funding

Funding for the evaluative research was provided by NHS England.

Notes

1. The National Health Service is the publicly funded national healthcare system for England.
2. https://en.unesco.org/youth
3. Exists to protect and improve the nation's health and wellbeing and reduce health inequalities.
4. Now the Department of Health and Social Care, responsible for government policy on health and adult social care matters in England.
5. Clinically led statutory NHS bodies responsible for the planning and commissioning of healthcare services for their local area.
6. www.facebook.com/NHSEnglandYF/
7. www.england.nhs.uk/participation/get-involved/how/forums/nhs-youth-forum/
8. www.gosh.nhs.uk/teenagers/teengosh-community/young-peoples-forum/big-youth-forum-meet
9. www.youtube.com/watch?v=FU-52Dxmf3g
10. www.england.nhs.uk/contact-us/complaint/
11. www.england.nhs.uk/participation/get-involved/how/forums/nhs-youth-forum/
12. www.youtube.com/watch?v=sBSA_8hQEmA
13. www.byc.org.uk/wp-content/uploads/2018/01/BYC-NHS-Transition-v2.pdf
14. www.youngpeopleshealth.org.uk/
15. www.england.nhs.uk/new-care-models/
16. www.iwill.org.uk/
17. bwc.nhs.uk/volunteering-roles
18. www.sexualhealthsheffield.nhs.uk/get-involved/pash-project/
19. Ensures that the NHS workforce has the appropriate skills to deliver safe and effective high-quality care.
20. Regulates and inspects health and social care services in England.
21. Expo inspires leaders and clinicians to make improvements for patients and service users.

References

Aspland, D. (2015) What does participation look like? A circle or a ladder? Available from: www.specialneedsjungle.com/what-does-participation-look-like-a-circle-or-a-ladder/ [Last accessed: 17th February 2020].

Blackpool Teaching Hospitals NHS Foundation Trust (2018) *Case study: Involving young patients in the teaching and induction of Doctors*. Available from: www.nhsemployers.org/~/media/Employers/Documents/Recruit/Children%20and%20Young%20People/Doctors%20induction%20top%20tips%20-%20Blackpool.pdf [Last accessed: 23rd April 2019].

BYC and NHS England (2017) NHS Youth Forum Activity & Impact Report 2013-17. Available from: https://www.england.nhs.uk/wp-content/uploads/2018/07/FINAL-Youth-Forum-Activity-Impact-Report-2013-to-2017.pdf [Last accessed: 21st May 2020].

CHF (Consumers Health Forum of Australia) (2018) *Inaugural youth health forum*. Available from: https://chf.org.au/events/inaugural-youth-health-forum [Last accessed: 24th April 2019].

Collins, M.E., Augsberger, A. and Gecker, W. (2016) Youth councils in municipal government: Examination of activities, impact and barriers. *Children and Youth Services Review*, 65, pp 140–7.

Creswell, J.W. (2012) *Educational Research: Planning, Conducting, and Evaluating Quantitative and Qualitative Research*. 4th edition. Boston: Pearson.

Department of Education and Science (1982) *Experience and participation. Review group on the youth service in England* ('The Thompson Report'). HMSO: London.

Hart, R.A. (1992) *Children's participation: From tokenism to citizenship*. Innocenti Research Centre. Florence: UNICEF.

Matthews, H. (2001) Citizenship, youth councils and young people's participation. *Journal of Youth Studies*, 4 (3), pp 299–318.

Matthews, H. and Limb, M. (1998) The right to say: The development of youth councils/forums within the UK. *Area*, 30 (1), pp 66–78.

Moule, P. and Goodman, M. (2014) *Nursing Research: An Introduction*. 2nd edition. London: Sage Publications Ltd.

NHS England (2015a) *NHS England and the British Youth Council. Bitesize guide to setting up a youth forum in health services across England*. Available from: www.england.nhs.uk/wp-content/uploads/2015/02/how-to-guid-yth-forum.pdf [Last accessed: 23rd April 2019].

NHS England (2015b) *The NHS Constitution. The NHS belongs to us all.* Available from: https://assets.publishing.service.gov. uk/government/uploads/system/uploads/attachment_data/ file/480482/NHS_Constitution_WEB.pdf [Last accessed: 23rd April 2019].

NHS England (2016) *NHS Youth Forum youth rights in healthcare posters.* Available from: www.england.nhs.uk/participation/ get-involved/how/forums/nhs-youth-forum/ [Last accessed: 23rd April 2019].

Northern Ireland Youth Forum (2019) *About NIYF.* Available from: https://www.niyf.org/about-niyf/ [Last accessed: 23rd April 2019].

Office of National Statistics (2017) *Overview of the UK population: July 2017.* Available from: www.ons.gov.uk/peoplepopulation andcommunity/populationandmigration/populationestimates/ articles/overviewoftheukpopulation/july2017 [Last accessed: 23rd April 2019].

Office of the Children's Commissioner (2015) *Participation strategy June 2014-May 2015.* Available from: https://dera.ioe. ac.uk/20552/1/participation_strategy_2014_2015.pdf [Last accessed: 17th February 2020].

Royal College of Paediatrics and Child Health (RCPCH) (2017) *State of Child Health: Report 2017.* London: RCPCH. Available from: https://www.yhphnetwork.co.uk/media/1601/state-of-child-health-england-rcpch-2018.pdf [Last accessed: 23rd April 2019].

Salusky, I., Larson, R.L., Griffith, A., Wu, J., Raffaelli, M., Sugimura, N. and Guzman, M. (2014) How adolescents develop responsibility: What can be learned from youth programs. *Journal of Research on Adolescence,* 24 (3), pp 417–30.

Sherrod, L.R., Flanagan, C. and Youniss, J. (2002) Dimensions on citizenship and opportunities for youth development: The what, why, when, where, and who of citizenship development. *Applied Developmental Science,* 6 (4), pp 264–72.

United Nations Educational, Scientific and Cultural Organization (UNESCO) (2019) *UNESCO youth forum: By youth for youth.* Available fromhttps://www.un.org/en/sections/resources-different-audiences/students/index.html [Last accessed: 23rd April 2019].

Whiting, L., Roberts, S., Meager, G. and Petty, J. (2016a) *An examination of the work of the National Health Service [NHS] England Youth Forum.* Hatfield: University of Hertfordshire. Available from: http://researchprofiles.herts. ac.uk/portal/files/10549906/An_examination_of_the_work_ of_the_National_Health_Service_NHS_England_Youth_ Forum_11.10.16_both_logos.pdf [Last accessed: 26th April 2019].

Whiting, L., Roberts, S., Etchells, J., Evans, K. and Williams, A. (2016b) An evaluation of the NHS England Youth Forum. *Nursing Standard, Art & Science,* 31 (2), pp 45–53.

Whiting, L., Roberts, S., Petty, J., Meager, G. and Evans, K. (2018) Work of the NHS England Youth Forum and its effect on health services. *Nursing Children and Young People,* 30 (4), pp 34–40.

Wyness, M. (2009) Adult's Involvement in children's participation: Juggling children's places and spaces. *Children & Society,* 23 (6), pp 395–406.

Youth Forum (1999) The next step. Youth forum. *Integration,* 60, pp 9–10.

Appendix 3.1

University of
Hertfordshire

An examination of the work
of the NHS England Youth Forum
Activity Log

Name: _____ Age: _____

Gender (please tick)   Male [ ]   Female [ ]

Home (please specify your town/village and area in England (for example, Hatfield, Hertfordshire:

_____

Day to day activity (For example, school, college, University, work, volunteer):

_____

Membership of any other organisations or Youth Forums (for example, Youth Parliament – please name):

NHS England Youth Forum activity (please describe)	In which capacity are doing this activity?	Date	Length of time	Where	Cost

4

RCPCH &Us: improving healthcare through engagement

Emma Sparrow and Mike Linney

Introduction

The Royal College of Paediatrics and Child Health (RCPCH) Children and Young People's Engagement Team works to ensure that the voice of children, young people and families is used to improve health care for young patients. RCPCH &Us, launched in April 2015, have engaged with over 7,000 children, young people and families up until January 2020, with 1,000 professional members of their Engagement Collaborative.

Box 4.1: RCPCH definition of CYP

Children and young people (CYP) – are defined by the RCPCH Engagement Committee as infants, children, young people and their advocates: parents, carers, families, friends, healthcare professionals, support workers, plus others.

Royal College of Paediatrics and Child Health (RCPCH) (2020)

This chapter explores how the 'RCPCH &Us' network and Engagement Collaborative actively seeks and shares the views of children, young people and families to influence and shape health policy and practice. This includes examples of consultation, engagement and co-production with children and young people (CYP) creating a new approach to sharing information, informing standards, improving understanding and creating better services.

RCPCH &Us: educate, collaborate, engage and change. Improving the quality of healthcare by engagement and collaboration

'Close your eyes. Think of your biggest secret.... Think of the one that makes you feel sick in your stomach. Keep thinking. How would you feel if I told you to tell a room of strangers your secret? This is how infants, children and young people can sometimes feel about health. In the dark and afraid, not sure if the person they are going to tell will understand their secret or be able to help them.' Takeover Challenge[1] RCPCH &Us Wales young people, 2016

Figure 4.1: Our right to health by RCPCH &Us, 2017

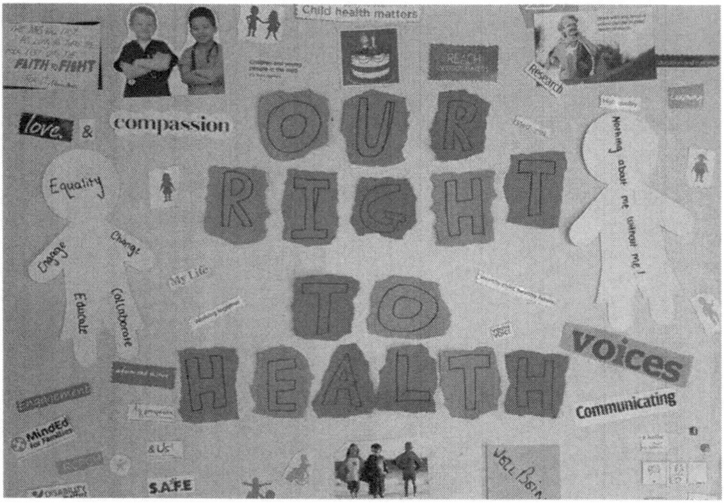

Source: Ball (2017)

Being in the dark about appointments, discussions, policymaking and decision-making is a challenge for most children and young people we have worked with. Our aim is to make sure that everyone feels they are informed, consulted, involved and represented in healthcare policy and practice.

The health of infants and CYP is at the core of everything that the RCPCH[2] does. We ensure every paediatrician has the knowledge and expertise to promote child health and to care for infants, children and young people with health needs. We continue to improve the health and wellbeing of infants, children and young people in the UK and across the world through campaigning, advocacy, research, global programmes to improve healthcare in developing countries, education, training and continuous professional development for paediatricians.

RCPCH has developed an innovative approach to involving children and young people in shaping health policy and practice. RCPCH &Us was established in April 2015 to ensure that the voice of children, young people and families makes a difference in the work of RCPCH, the child health sector and in healthcare services and policies for young patients. This chapter will focus on our programmes with young people and how they are involved at a UK level to work with the NHS so that they have access to the best healthcare possible.

Our work includes projects, events, activities and sharing news to educate, collaborate, engage and change services for the better.

Figure 4.2: RCPCH &Us Logo, 2018

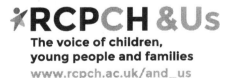

Source: RCPCH (2018)

The RCPCH &Us Network includes:

- **RCPCH &Us News** through our social media channels and a monthly e-newsletter;

- **RCPCH &Us Roadshows** across the UK to find out what children and young people from all ages and backgrounds think about child health topics;
- **RCPCH &Us Challenges** bringing together groups of children, young people and/or parents and carers for the day to work together on a topic, review the Roadshow information and come up with ideas and solutions;
- **RCPCH &Us Projects** where children, young people and families get involved over a longer time to work on turning ideas into products and developing new solutions to challenges;
- **RCPCH &Us Represent** where children, young people and families are supported to share the platform with the decision makers, representing the views of the wider network to inform, influence and lobby for change.

Since its launch in 2015:

- over 7,000 children, young people and family members have shared their voices, views, needs and wishes and health topics;
- over 4,000 healthcare workers have been in sessions exploring the RCPCH model for engagement;
- 1,000 workers have joined the Engagement Collaborative supporting workers on how to involve children and young people in shaping services;
- over 360 young people and family members have signed up to join the RCPCH &Us Network.

Our approach

Strategic voice

The focus of RCPCH &Us is to work with children, young people, families, RCPCH members (paediatricians), health services and decision makers on improving the 'strategic voice' of children and young people within the NHS. This refers to supporting and enabling collective groups of children and young people to work at a strategic, service-wide level through meaningful engagement and participation approaches.

Figure 4.3: What is strategic voice? Engagement Collaborative, 2017

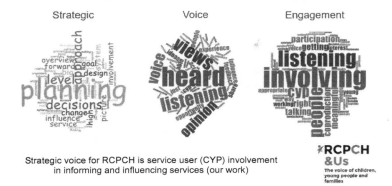

Strategic voice for RCPCH is service user (CYP) involvement in informing and influencing services (our work)

Source: RCPCH (2017)

Strategic voice, where RCPCH service users (children and young people) are involved in informing and influencing services and our work within the NHS and child health settings, is important in order for services to meet the needs of their service users.

Within the NHS, emphasis is placed on the strategic voice: *service users coming together to shape services with staff.* The NHS Constitution (2013)[3] makes it clear that patients and the public have the right to be involved in the planning of healthcare services commissioned by NHS bodies, the development and consideration of proposals for changes affecting the operation of those services. This is legislated through section 242(1B)[4] of the National Health Service Act 2006 as amended by the Local Government & Public Involvement in Health Act 2007. This includes the work and services of Clinical Commissioning Groups and NHS England.

Exploration of the policy and legislative drivers for strategic voice across the UK can be found in the RCPCH Engagement Legislation briefing (2017).[5]

Children and young people are at the centre of the RCPCH strategic plan (see Figure 4.4) which ensures that across the College, teams and divisions consider the impact of their work on children and young people, and work with the Engagement Team to develop meaningful opportunities to inform or influence this work.

Figure 4.4: RCPCH strategic plan, 2018

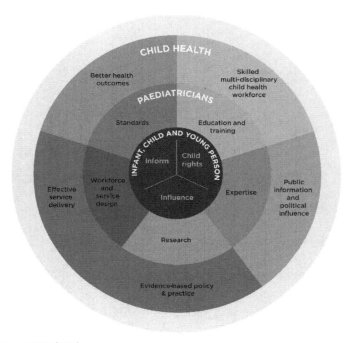

Source: RCPCH (2020)

The theory behind our approach falls into four different engagement areas of work:

- **educate** children and young people of their rights and responsibilities, the opportunities available to them to engage (RCPCH &Us News) and to share their voices and views with decision makers;
- **collaborate with** the voice and views of children and young people on a range of child health topics alongside healthcare professionals (RCPCH &Us Roadshows/Challenges/Projects);
- **engage** children and young people to create and lead solutions through projects and child or youth led initiatives (RCPCH &Us Challenges/Projects);
- **change** policy and practice through active involvement and influence at decision-making forums with children and young people (RCPCH &Us Represent).

The approach draws from theories including 'degrees of participation' (Tresder, 1997), 'archetypes of participation' (Kaizen Partnership Ltd, 2013), empowerment (Rowlands, 1997), anti oppressive and anti discriminatory practice (Thompson, 2006; Chouhan, 2009), 'The Art of Consultation' (Jones and Gammell, 2009).

Diversity and inclusion

Throughout our work we have an inclusive approach to engagement, ensuring that we keep in mind that our service users are children and young people first, users of health services second. We are proud of our diverse working practices which ensure diverse children and young people can take part in a way that is appropriate to their needs, for example using communication aids, working with advocates and support workers or families, developing bespoke materials to meet a variety of communication, physical, sensory or learning needs.

We have developed a voice diversity model which is used in all our work, from RCPCH &Us Roadshows to challenge days to project sessions. We look to go where children and young people are based, reducing their travel and working with them in settings where they feel comfortable and at ease. We also aim to include the voices and views of children and young people from the following backgrounds:

- **universal voices** accessed through open access sessions where having a health experience is not a necessity, for example schools, youth clubs, summer holiday schemes;
- **targeted voices** where there is something that unites children and young people or there is a common experience that brings them together, for example hospital patients forum, looked after children's forum, young carers project;
- **specialist voices** where we are looking for a specific condition or health experience, for example speaking with patients in a clinic, chats at a teen cancer chemo outpatient unit or epilepsy clinic.

Box 4.2: RCPCH &Us voice diversity model, 2016

Voice diversity = universal + targeted + specialist voices

RCPCH, 2017

By accessing the voices and views of all three groups, we can triangulate their ideas and experiences, guarding against bias, for example where a universal young person has no experience of an outpatient clinic or where a child has been in and out of hospital for years offering an institutionalised response.

It all starts with rights!

> 'How many of you have heard of the United Nations Convention on the Rights of the Child (UNCRC)?[6] How many of you can name at least ten of the articles and why they are important for children and young people?' RCPCH &Us Member, Scott

This question is the starting point for all our sessions, discussions and presentations about RCPCH &Us, engagement or participation in health services. The UNCRC covers all aspects of a child's life and sets out the civil, political, economic, social and cultural rights that children everywhere are entitled to.

Figure 4.5: RCPCH &Us voice bank

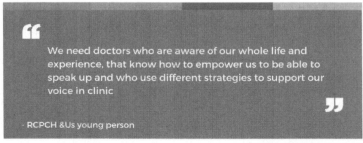

> "We need doctors who are aware of our whole life and experience, that know how to empower us to be able to speak up and who use different strategies to support our voice in clinic"
>
> - RCPCH &Us young person

#VoiceMatters

⚡RCPCH &Us
The voice of children,
young people and families

Source: RCPCH (2017)

Having a rights-based approach[7] for RCPCH &Us means that we take seriously our role in supporting children and young people's dignity, participation, development, non-discrimination and best interests within strategic voice in health, their right to interdependence and indivisibility and our role in being transparent and accountable across their engagement.

RCPCH &Us young people have discussed and prioritised for action the following five articles within our work in NHS and child health services, with an acknowledgement that all articles are as important as each other and are fundamental for children and young people to have a safe and supported childhood.

- **Article 12** – right for children and young people to be involved in decisions that affect them, from individual care decisions through to shaping health services that they might use;
- **Article 23** – children and young people with disabilities have the right to be involved, which includes having appropriate communication support within health care appointments and engagement work;

Figure 4.6: Article 12, RCPCH 21st birthday, 2017

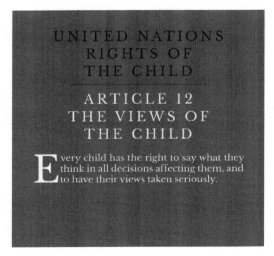

Source: Ball (2017)

- **Article 24** – the right to the best healthcare possible, including child- and youth-friendly health services;
- **Article 28** – the right to education, thinking about while they are an inpatient, or structuring services to avoid missing school due to medical appointments or supporting engagement sessions in evening and weekends/school holidays;
- **Article 31** – the right to rest, relax and play which in a health context also needs to include support for parents of children with complex health needs to think about how to engage in social activities, and for healthcare services to acknowledge their role in providing services that don't prevent children and young people from socialising with their peers (for example clinic times).

In 2016, we worked with groups of children, young people and families across the UK to find out what they thought were the fundamental rights for the best healthcare possible. As part of the Facing the Future[8] programme, young patients and their families told us that it was about having the right time, the right place, the right people and knowing their rights.[9]

Figure 4.7: Article 24, RCPCH 21st birthday, 2017

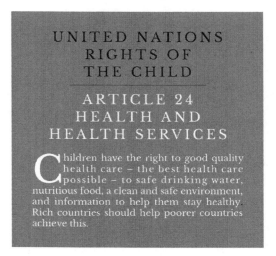

Source: Ball (2017)

Embedding RCPCH &Us into practice

How do we embed the voice of service users into practice, what have we learnt and what difference does it make? We have highlighted examples of new approaches developed within RCPCH, exploring the challenges, solutions created by our young volunteers, learning and comments from children, young people or family members involved.

Figure 4.8: RCPCH &Us voice bank

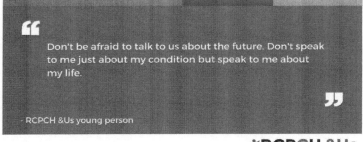

Source: RCPCH (2017)

Box 4.3: Challenge one: lack of evidence of what children and young people voice

Collating comments from children and young people on what they think, feel, need or hope for within child health services/the NHS is challenging at a national level. Ensuring it is extensive in geographical and demographical reach, that it includes live rather than historical data and that it goes on to support thinking for those creating policy, standards and guidelines for the NHS can prove problematic.

The solution: develop the RCPCH &Us Roadshow model where staff visit children and young people at their location, in a range of universal, targeted and specialist settings across the UK, to take opportunities to them to inform and influence policy and practice. All consultation responses are stored in a 'voice bank' which is then used as a repository for views on child health/NHS services.

The learning: patients and their families are very keen to share their ideas, comments and views, but how this is done needs to adapt to cohort needs. Visiting them in clinics (waiting room clinic chats) or through schools and youth settings supports their engagement, provides an endorsement through their trusted service or worker and allows them to engage face to face rather than through a survey or questionnaire. Non-engagement specialists need support to learn how to interact in this way, using anti oppressive practice and archetypes of participation approaches cited previously to support good quality engagement approaches.

What our stakeholders said: "Having the RCPCH &Us Voice Bank means my voice is captured forever, it allows me to support the team and the RCPCH in different ways rather than re-treading old ground. Through the RCPCH &Us Voice Bank, I am able to influence, use my voice to strength[en] others and substantiate claims/outputs from the College. It allows for a wider breadth of voice to be collected as opposed to only having a chosen few who always get to comment. The RCPCH &Us Voice Bank really harnesses the diversity of the voice model and really upholds the principal of going to where young people are and collecting feedback/voice at a time that is right for them and in a place they would be anyway. It is not just collection for collection's sake."

Box 4.4: Challenge two: embedding children and young people's voice in child health governance

Creating approaches for top-level representative roles on committees, programme boards and as trustees in a consistent and meaningful way can be a challenge. There are elements to overcome such as logistical issues including timing of meetings, language used, depth of knowledge needed and cultural changes around meeting format, style and accessibility.

The solution: RCPCH has developed a new committee structure called 'The CYP Engagement Committee' and reshaped the engagement model around committee voice. The CYP Engagement Committee is delivered through a workshop approach with a committee membership which includes children, young people and parents alongside paediatricians and voluntary sector representatives. Within other committees and representative bodies, voice is collated and shared by advocates, projects are developed and delivered out of committee meeting with children and young people, and champions are supported in committees to liaise between service users and committee representatives. The RCPCH Guidance for chairs, committee members and staff (2018)[10] shares the challenges and identifies solutions to ensure there is appropriate, meaningful, proportionate and relevant engagement opportunities.

The learning: it has taken a great deal of support and time to develop the 'voice in committees' model in a way that supports the drive to have 'lay representatives' round the table to a more meaningful engagement response. Where RCPCH committees or NHS Trust boards meet during the school day, using a traditional meeting style, the cultural change needed has required support, challenge and the use of an 'appreciative inquiry' approach (Martins, 2014).

What our stakeholders said: "The review of lay members on College Committees by the CYP Engagement Committee ensured that all involvement in committees is not tokenistic and is facilitated in the most appropriate way for CYP representatives to feed into priorities and work of committees. The Engagement Committee is a revolutionary way of doing governance and influencing a Charity/Health Sector/Programmes, children and young people very much leading the way in engagement at RCPCH and in strategy through Trustee role, children and young people were involved in the recruitment of the Chief Executive, Beneficiary Trustee, Chair of Trustees, Trustee Board Member Representatives + External Representatives with children and young people's influence and value shown throughout. I feel far more empowered, valued through new way[s] of engaging with governance at the RCPCH. I feel that it is far more impactful and we get more achieved. It's all about what gets done rather than what we just talk about! Results! Not just hot air!"

You can find out more about this best practice model produced by RCPCH &Us at the Plan, Do, Study and Act case study on QI Central (www.qicentral.org.uk).

Box 4.5: Challenge three: voice and influence in national audit programmes

Supporting children and young people to have influence in national audit programmes within the NHS is complex and often not linked to their role in auditing and improving practice nationally. Traditionally, national audits are incredibly data heavy, with clinicians inputting huge volumes of individual patient data into a national repository, which is then analysed and data published 12–18 months after data entry, to identify areas for quality improvement. While data from children, young people and families are generally included in audits their influence is often restricted to roles within committees for 1 or 2 'lay members' (usually parents).

The solution: the Epilepsy12 Audit is in its third cycle (each one being three years), assigning funds to develop a youth-led project where young people review the needs of children and young people with epilepsy and their families, then develop their own youth-led solutions. In 2018, over 130 patients and families shared their ideas through clinic chats, which were thematically analysed by the Epilepsy12 Youth Advocates for key themes. This has been developed into a youth-led project focusing on 'helping epilepsy patients and families with their worries and anxieties relating to epilepsy' which includes a unit self-assessment of support available, visits by youth advocates to co-produce an action plan with a follow-up visit six months later. The engagement project has recently won a national award from HQIP (2018) for patient involvement in audits recognising the work of the E12 Youth Advocates.

The learning: working within a data-heavy system is challenging to identify meaningful opportunities for children and young people that provide opportunities to influence and see outputs in a realistic timeframe for patients. The development of a quality improvement project led by young people which meets their needs and builds in success relating to their personal development is important. Having good project outputs and epilepsy care outcomes also helps to unite patient and families with the audit programme while providing a supportive resource for units providing epilepsy care.

What our stakeholders said: "Sometimes living with an invisible illness, it can seem that seizures are unstoppable. But looking at the results of the clinic chats, the children and young people are the ones who are unstoppable. My wish for Epilepsy12 going forward is for practitioners to engage further with young people about their treatment, especially as patients start to grow up and come up to that transition. I would strongly recommend children, young people, siblings, families, clinicians, specialist nurses and other paediatricians as well as other engagement groups should all come together and be made aware of what has been said. This way we can put forward an agenda and help shape the future of Epilepsy12 and other audits promoting children and young people, their rights and their wellness."

You can read more about this national award-winning project in the HQIP case study www.hqip.org.uk/resource/case-study-epilepsy12/# and the youth advocates Epilepsy12 Report www.rcpch.ac.uk/resources/epilepsy12-us-voices-rcpch-us-network.

Box 4.6: Challenge four: voice in the training and assessment of paediatricians

Children and young people are the centre of everything we do at RCPCH. It's important that within paediatric curriculum design, clinical exams, continuous professional development and consultant assessments, children and young people also have a formative role in the process. With children and young people involved in exams being all ages, in all locations across the UK, there is a challenge around how you develop a process that is rights-based, formative, child/young people-focused and supportive for trainee paediatricians.

The solution: over a three-year period, we worked with the Education and Training Division, paediatricians, children, young people and families to understand where they would like to be involved and to develop appropriate engagement projects. RCPCH &Us Roadshows took place to identify 'what makes the best paediatrician' to inform the new curriculum launched in 2018. RCPCH &Us Challenges and Projects took place looking at developing emoji assessment tools for clinical exams giving patients the chance to share their formative assessment on how the trainee doctor communicated and built rapport, with other workshops that took place with young people to develop consultant assessment scenarios on youth issues.

The learning: working within paediatric training is incredibly complex in relation to the curriculum, exam structures, red tape and extensive reach across the UK and to global exam centres in Egypt, United Arab Emirates, India and others, plus the balance between being child- and young person-focused in approach and keeping the trainee paediatrician in mind. Through having good stakeholder involvement with robust stakeholder mapping, there has been engagement throughout the process with key partners like the GMC, clinical examiners, trainees, patients and their families which have supported the development of the programme. Being challenged on the 'why, how and what' has helped to refine messaging, to understand each other's points of view and to remain outcome-focused – to create the best paediatrician possible. Children and young people want to support us on this journey, but to deliver this strategically we have to move past projects and embed into systems – in this case the curriculum used in training paediatricians and their exam process.

What our stakeholders said: the best doctor is ... "informed about national & local services support for children and young people, signposting and engaging with them." When I visit my doctor about my gastroenterology condition, I would like... "to see pictures and stories of other children living well with what I have". "When we leave an emergency department, we need to be given clear and easy to understand verbal and written information (or are transferred) so we know what to do when we get home or if something changes. Take time to find out who we are not just what is wrong. It is important that doctors know about things that affect children and help us to talk about things that may not be easy like mental health. We need doctors that can empower us and use different strategies in clinic to hear our voice".

You can read more about this at www.rcpch.ac.uk/education-careers/ training/progress, and published by the *BMJ* www.bmj.com/content/ 361/bmj.k1829. The patients who decide what makes a good doctor, *BMJ* 2018.

Impact of our approach in embedding strategic voice in the NHS

The key question for our work is… *so what?* It's one that we asked members of the CYP Engagement Committee and they said:

Personal impact of being involved in strategic voice programmes:

- "It has made me feel more empowered. Before I joined RCPCH &Us, I was very isolated, quiet and mildly depressed. Joining the network really made me feel for the first time that I had power in my own life. I felt that my voice and experience was important and could affect change. For the first time, I felt that I could use all my experiences, good and bad, to inform and improve care for other young people like me going through the NHS in the future."
- "Meeting other young people who are as passionate about health and their health, made me feel really connected and like I was no longer alone. The strength and bond created through the network has really made me feel fulfilled."
- "The skills and opportunities I have gained through the network have made me a much more well-rounded individual. I have improved my public speaking massively. When I was 15, I broke down in tears when asked to speak in front of my classmates for two minutes, but now I am quite happy taking on a room full of thousands of paediatricians/GPs/ policymakers/stakeholders and share my own experience, give suggestions of how to collaboratively work to improve the situation and build positive relations."

They also considered the **impact on the wider community of young patients and their families**:

- "The work of RCPCH has allowed patients to feel more connected and that their issues are not isolated and that they are not alone."

- "Given voice to the entirety of four nations. Not just isolated to major cities within those four nations but far flung (rural + urban)."
- "Empowering and skilling up young people that may not have had opportunity otherwise. Giving them connections, networks and skills to allow them to pursue their passions while also giving useful insight which allows for general improvement of healthcare system."
- "Patient representatives are truly valued as part of RCPCH &Us, and their views and ideas are used to make sustained impact. The emphasis has moved from simply talking to young people to see what they think but to actively involving them in designing training, resources and policies."

Finally, they thought about **how this work has an impact on the sector strategically**:

- "RCPCH is able to draw on an existing bank of good methods of engagement and uses that alongside developing new and innovative ways with young people. Not reinventing the wheel but modernising it and really consolidating co-ownership and co-production with children and young people."
- "Empowerment and giving real power to young people is the way forward."
- "RCPCH &Us has taken this one step further through creating the 'recipes for engagement' to inform health and social care professionals on how to engage, again using children and young people as the focal informant. This means that good practice is spread far and wide and not just carried out in silos (as so often is the case in healthcare). There is still a long way to go, however, as past paediatric patient, current adult patient and future healthcare professional, I hope the values that RCPCH &Us promotes will be second nature before too long."
- "I've also learnt an enormous amount [of] meaningful (and incredibly productive!) engagement from witnessing engagement in action in the innovative way that the committee meetings are chaired. This has allowed me to

be a much more effective champion for strategic voice of children and young people and given me the confidence to constructively challenge when I think more could be done to ensure their involvement in decision-making (in the commissioning of services as well as at service delivery level)."

Future development for strategic voice in the NHS

We asked RCPCH &Us children, young people, families, RCPCH members (paediatricians) and the Engagement Collaborative (wider sector staff) what they would like to see developed over the next few years in relation to voice, engagement and active involvement of children and young people shaping services and they said:

RCPCH &Us want RCPCH to:
- "continue to be leaders in good participation and engagement work";
- "continue working with a wide range of partners to learn best practice, continue to develop recipes for engagement techniques with children and young people to ensure they are current and meet their needs";
- "CYP to stay at the heart of RCPCH and everything it does";

Figure 4.9: RCPCH &Us voice bank

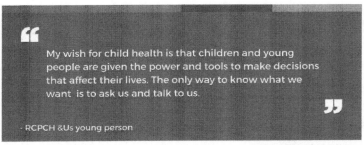

My wish for child health is that children and young people are given the power and tools to make decisions that affect their lives. The only way to know what we want is to ask us and talk to us.

- RCPCH &Us young person

#VoiceMatters

⚕RCPCH &Us
The voice of children,
young people and families

Source: Ball (2017)

- "CYP are supported in assessing/auditing reviewing all relevant services to them and giving their focused recommendations for improvement";
- "engagement toolkit to be produced that can be used by the entire sector, using all good learnings from Engagement Collaborative, CYP Engagement Committee and the Team's wider work".

RCPCH &Us think the wider sector should:
- "ensure engagement with CYP becomes commonplace and as part of business as usual for all involved and working in children and young people's health";
- "be consistent as to what engagement and participation means to all involved with working with and for children and young people";
- "have real, practical involvement for children and young people across the country and the world. Getting children, young people and their families centre stage when it comes to planning their care and in delivery";
- "children and young people becoming their own advocates[11] if possible, with the right support right across the board";
- "my hope for the next few years is that commissioners[12] and regulators at a local and national level fully understand the importance of engagement. Children and young people's voice needs to inform decisions about allocation of resources and defining what a high-quality service looks like";
- "my hope for the future is that the voice of children and young people is heard and understood by senior managers at all levels (from individual hospitals and GP practices to regional and national commissioning and regulatory bodies)".

RCPCH members (paediatricians)

Throughout 2018, the CYP Engagement Committee worked with members and an external researcher to review what support is needed to increase engagement by children and young people in the child health sector. This provided insights into why members do or do not currently engage with children and young people in service design or strategic voice projects such as the Epilepsy12 Youth Advocates project highlighted previously. Members would like to do a lot more engagement and would like more support (see further on for suggestions) to be able to do so. Time to engage well across a range of levels and approaches, with appropriate resources such as staff time, project budgets to cover travel, materials and specialist staff, for example youth workers/interpreters are the biggest barriers for members to do more engagement which needs to be considered when designing solutions to support them.

It is also clear that perceptions of the senior management teams and commissioners need to be influenced about the importance and impact that engagement with children and young people has on service design. Ensuring they:

- are aware of the resources needed to develop a meaningful engagement programme;
- how to develop programmes using the rights-based approach, where we start from where the child or young person is at rather than the data need of a service;
- are clear on where and how engagement voices will feed into decision-making structures such as trust board, senior management team meetings, programme boards.

Thinking through these three areas in advance, with robust conversations between engagement specialists, clinicians, commissioners and patients will support engagement programmes to have more influence and success in shaping services and informing policy and practice.

Finally, the research demonstrates the importance that the RCPCH &Us team has in supporting members in children and young people's engagement. The responses received demonstrated the desire for further access to the Engagement Team at RCPCH and to have local dedicated resources in terms of skilled staff to take strategic voice and engagement forward.

In addition to this work, the 2018 RCPCH member survey also offered a chance for over 1,800 RCPCH members from across the UK, at different stages in their specialist paediatric training or as consultant paediatricians, to share views on *what support with engagement would be beneficial to your role?*

Their responses included:

- children and young people's assessments of services/peer reviews: 55 per cent;
- children and young people's voice reports on child health topics: 41 per cent;
- training on setting up an engagement programme: 39 per cent;
- toolkits about engagement: 36 per cent;
- coaching/mentoring: 35 per cent;
- training on children's rights: 28 per cent.

Figure 4.10: RCPCH member's survey, 2018

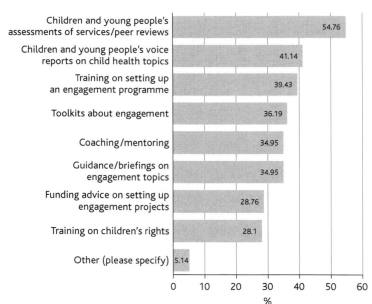

Source: RCPCH (2018)

Engagement Collaborative members

Throughout 2018, over 100 Engagement Collaborative members took part in *The Art and Science of Effective Engagement with Children and Young People*[13] training courses, led by the Kaizen Partnership Ltd[14] on behalf of RCPCH. This course looked at what engagement is, how to develop an engagement plan and how to ensure your approach meets the needs of a diverse range of service users and has impact within your setting. Attendees shared their views on what was needed in the future to continue to support engagement:

- online resource kits;
- time and resources;
- practical examples of best practice;
- to integrate this into their role;
- senior colleague buy in and support;
- train the trainer materials.

Conclusion

RCPCH &Us with the support of the wider Royal College staff group and membership body of paediatricians, is central to the future of engagement in health services for children and young people. Over the coming years, there will be a focus on increasing the scope and influence of strategic voice in three key areas:

- training and assessment of paediatricians;
- shaping health policy;
- supporting our workforce to increase knowledge, skills and confidence in engagement practice determined from the ideas, views and needs of children, young people, families and the sector.

It is clear from the views of our stakeholders explored in the last section, RCPCH &Us children, young people and their families, RCPCH members (paediatricians) and Engagement Collaborative members (wider sector professionals) that there is a real energy and passion around engagement in the health sector. There are common themes emerging that the sector has to consider in order to support challenges relating to participation and engagement. These are:

- develop opportunities for children and young people to have a role in shaping and auditing services at a national, regional and local level;
- develop/promote existing engagement toolkits, voice reports and practical resources to support advocacy, campaigning and championing the strategic voice in shaping services;
- everyone to be accountable and responsible for embedding voice as commonplace and business as usual for all involved, following the UNCRC and statutory guidance for the NHS;
- increase confidence through training, information sharing/ networking, advice and guidance on engagement practice.

RCPCH, in its aim to lead in transforming child health through innovation, influence, leadership and inclusion extends to having a strong RCPCH &Us programme. This keeps children and young people at the centre of everything we do. Our work programmes will continue to involve children and young people in shaping services:

- workforce development with young people running training sessions for paediatricians;
- extend our youth advocates model in national audit programmes;
- ensure policy, standards and guidelines by RCPCH are informed by the voices and views of children and young people.

Children and young people have to be involved in child health services to ensure they are future proofed and meet their needs. RCPCH &Us delivers this through its principles of educate, collaborate, engage and change, and looks forward to this continuing to inform and influence health policy and practice across the UK.

Acknowledgments

We would like to thank the following people from the CYP Engagement Committee, who made invaluable contributions to the development and drafting of this chapter: Thines Ganeshamoorthy and Charlotte Underwood (RCPCH &Us representatives), Lynn Hoppenbrouwers (voluntary sector representative), Carmen Soto and Rebecca Hewitson (RCPCH member representatives), Hana Najsrova (RCPCH staff member).

Notes

1. www.childrenscommissioner.gov.uk/takeover-challenge/
2. www.rcpch.ac.uk/resources/rcpch-annual-review
3. www.gov.uk/government/publications/the-nhs-constitution-for-england
4. www.legislation.gov.uk/ukpga/2006/41/contents
5. www.rcpch.ac.uk/sites/default/files/And_Us_-_Legislation_briefing.pdf
6. www.unicef.org.uk/what-we-do/un-convention-child-rights/
7. www.unicef.org.uk/child-friendly-cities/child-rights-based-approach/
8. www.rcpch.ac.uk/resources/facing-future-standards-paediatric-care
9. https://youtu.be/E3303esR3Js
10. https://www.rcpch.ac.uk/sites/default/files/2018-04/involving_children_and_young_people_committees.pdf
11. www.rcpch.ac.uk/hiddenhealth_Parents at Alder Hey Children's Hospital have produced a guide with RCPCH &Us that supports this approach called 'Hidden Health'.
12. www.qicentral.org.uk/patient-centred-care/voices-and-views/involving-children-and-young-people-specialised-commissioning_A series of recommendations and solutions developed by young people with complex health needs to support commissioners in their ongoing work. You can access the full plan, do, study, act case study and resources from QI Central.
13. Kaizen Partnership Ltd (2018) *The Art and Science of Effective Engagement with Children and Young People.*
14. http://wearekaizen.co.uk/

References

Ball, J. (2017) *RCPCH: The First Twenty One Years.* London: RCPCH.

Chouhan, J. (2009) Anti-oppressive practice. In J. Wood and J. Hine (eds.) *Work with Young People.* London: Sage.

Jones, R. and Gammell, E. (2009) *The Art of Consultation.* London: Biteback Publishing.

Kaizen Partnership Ltd (2013) cited in *Kaizen Engagement Models: Engagement Strategy and Planning 2017.* London: Kaizen Partnership.

Kaizen Partnership Ltd (2018) *The Art and Science of Effective Engagement with Children and Young People.* https://prezi.com/jsho4b5iboxy/rcpch-nov-2018-roadshow/?token=ed7135bc6bcf205ae6796c86f65beb398a82d94bc85408c75a85020cb20258fb

Martins, C. (2014) *Appreciative Inquiry in Child Protection – Identifying and Promoting Good Practice and Creating a Learning Culture: Practice Tool.* Totnes: Research in Practice.

RCPCH (2017) https://www.rcpch.ac.uk/work-we-do/rcpch-us-children-young-people-families

RCPCH (2018) www.rcpch.ac.uk/and_us

RCPCH (2020) https://www.rcpch.ac.uk/

Rowlands, J. (1997) *Questioning Empowerment*. Oxford: Oxfam Publications.

Thompson, N. (2006) *Anti Discriminatory Practice*. 4th edition. Milton Keynes: Open University Press.

Tresder, P. (1997) *Empowering Children and Young People – Training Manual: Promoting Involvement in Decision-Making*. London: Save the Children.

5

Innovative ways of engaging young people whose voices are less heard

*Lindsay Starbuck, Kirsche Walker, Jack Welch,
Emma Rigby and Ann Hagell*

Introduction

The Association for Young People's Health (AYPH) is the UK's leading independent voice for youth health. We work to improve the health and wellbeing of 10–24-year-olds by improving understanding of young people's health needs and promoting youth-friendly health services. We do this through influencing policy and practice, producing evidence-based reports and briefings (such as our biennial *Key Data on Young People* publications), and running projects to test new models of health care delivery for this age group. Involving young people in all our activities is essential for us, and much of our work focuses on ensuring their voices are heard. AYPH has a particular mission to ensure that opportunities to engage in the development of health services are extended to young people who may be more marginalised from the mainstream, and who may find it harder to get their voices heard.

In this chapter we draw on three projects we have undertaken recently, each presenting rather different challenges to participation. The first was a project to get young people's views on acute care, the second related to young people who had been affected by sexual exploitation and the third was on obesity. Each presented different challenges relating to the particular topic of the study and the method of engagement, but there were also common lessons to be learned about how to engage more marginalised young people and how to draw on creative approaches to amplify their voices in ways that do not threaten their need for confidentiality. Two case studies from young people involved in participation projects illustrate some of these issues and their solutions.

Background

Every young person has a right to be heard. For those up to 18 this is enshrined in the UN Convention on the Rights of the Child (United Nations General Assembly, 1989). For those who are young adults the right may not be so clearly articulated in international protocols, but they have as much right as anyone else. This sounds obvious but is not always well articulated. In the UK, young people's participation in political and social dialogue is low (Electoral Commission, 2002; British Youth Council, 2015).

As well as being a fundamental right, having a voice is part of holding authorities and services to account, and this is a lever for improvement (NHS Institute for Innovation and Improvement, 2013; Crowley, 2015). Every young person has individual views based on their lived experiences and can never truly represent all young people. Young people who are marginalised – because of the nature of their trauma, illness or living circumstances – will have a unique perspective that can highlight how services may be perpetuating stigma, bias and discrimination. Actively seeking out the widest possible range of voices, especially those heard less often, is vital for developing health services that meet all young people's needs (World Health Organization [WHO], 2017).

Why is it more difficult to engage young people whose voices are less heard?

Although they may have extensive contact with health services, some groups of young people are less heard because of the particular challenges of their situation and the difficulties of finding ways to help them share their views (for example Berrick et al, 2000). Some young people are reluctant to come forward because they face considerable stigma and discrimination (YMCA/NHS, 2016). Some services work on the basis that young people who have experienced harm need more protection. Although this is clearly a good thing, it can also produce a risk averse environment where participation opportunities are not offered to young people (Coyne and Harder, 2011). There are a number of solutions to both of these issues. Those who are committed to involving young people need to strike a balance between protection and voice that recognises the right of all young people to be heard.

Stigma and discrimination

Involving young people who face stigma and/or discrimination because of their health conditions may require extra work and careful consideration on the part of those organising participation projects (Baker et al, 2014). Stigma can be perpetuated by other young people so it is not always possible for some young people to speak openly about their needs and experiences in mixed group activities. By developing opportunities where young people can work with others who have experienced similar oppression or trauma, participants are able to start from a place of acknowledging their shared problems and quickly move onto finding solutions together. Building up relationships and recruiting through specialist organisations where there is already trust and potentially an existing group is the most productive way to involve the most marginalised young people. Models which ensure the specialist organisation maintains an ongoing role are best as they can support more meaningful, longer-term engagement and participation. This ensures that young people have the support of an organisation that understands them and their experiences beyond the life of the project.

Perceived and real risks to young people

Young people who face stigma have a particular need for confidentiality and anonymity when they share their views or experiences (YMCA/NHS, 2016). For example, young people who are not living openly with their conditions or experiences cannot have their names included in publications, and any information that might reveal their identity or location has to be managed with extra care. If the aim of a project is to share the work publicly, young people need to give informed consent for this and be given the opportunity to define their identity as a group. This requires a high level of understanding of confidentiality, consent and risk on the part of everyone concerned (Heerman et al, 2015). The only way to manage issues around stigma and safeguarding in a way that meets the needs of marginalised young people is to work with them directly to decide what type of participation is best for them, both as individuals and as a group. For this reason, it is vital to have a youth-informed, flexible approach for every participation project that can accommodate and support young people with different needs (Rigby and Starbuck, 2018).

Engaging marginalised young people – practice examples

It is critically important that marginalised young people are heard so that services can be configured to meet their particular needs. In the long term, this can help them fulfil their potential and access the best possible healthcare. This section will outline three projects that AYPH has worked on that illustrate some of the challenges and potential solutions to involving marginalised groups of young people. We have included three quite different projects to demonstrate that it is possible to amplify marginalised young people's voices through a variety of approaches.

Acute Care project

AYPH was commissioned by the Royal College of Physicians (RCP) to run a participation project exploring acute care services with young people. The aim was to bring young people with different health experiences from two different regions of England together to create guidelines on working with young people in acute care settings. Although the RCP had existing resources on how to make acute care work for young people, adding youth voice was critical to making sure the messages were right. AYPH worked in partnership with specialist organisations who were already supporting young people around specific issues such as homelessness, physical disabilities and mental health, autism and HIV. Our partner projects included No Limits Southampton, Birmingham Sexual Health Service, Children's HIV Association (CHIVA), and Ambitious about Autism.

In the first stage, we ran focused workshops with 58 young people across both regions to find out their experiences of acute care and what they thought the barriers to using them were for their age group. For most of the groups, this involved a face-to-face meeting with AYPH's Youth Participation Coordinator who travelled to meet the young people in their own space, so that we could establish trusting relationships with the young people somewhere where they already felt comfortable. Twenty participants from these four services then met in London in January 2017 for a shared session. Together they created two brand-new youth-led resources about their experiences of acute care services and how those services can better meet the needs of all young people. The outputs included a short film highlighting the challenges of acute care settings and recommendations about how they could be improved (https://youtu.be/_5BGo7h9bpE). The project also resulted in AYPH's Acute Care flowchart (www.youngpeopleshealth.org.uk/acute-care-flowchart). The resources were complementary to the RCP's existing acute care toolkit for adolescents and young adults.

Be Healthy

Be Healthy was a long-term participation project run jointly by AYPH and the University of Bedfordshire's International Centre (www.ayph-behealthy.org.uk/). Three separate tranches of funding from Children in Need, Comic Relief and Big Lottery Awards for All supported the project from 2011 to 2015. A full account of the work is given in the project evaluation relating to the first tranche of funding (Hagell, 2013). The aim was to enable young people to highlight the unmet health needs of young people affected by child sexual exploitation (CSE) and develop resources for professionals on how to better support them. The definition of CSE used in the project included exploitative situations, contexts and relationships where young people receive something as a result of being part of sexual activities (DCSF, 2009; Barnardo's, 2012).

The project worked in partnership with three specialist CSE organisations in England, who each had existing trusted relationships with young people and could directly support their involvement. Ten young people worked with us intensively, some for up to three years or more. We worked locally and in small groups first, gradually moving to national large group meetings as trust and experience grew. Together the young people developed a host of resources about how to support and respect the agency of young people affected by CSE, including a website, animations and publications, which have been used by professionals in a variety of services and settings.

Promise

Promise was a research project conducted by University College London about the effectiveness of weight loss strategies for young people (www.ucl.ac.uk/promise). AYPH was asked to coordinate a young people's participation element in the final stages of the project in spring 2015. We developed an online survey that was completed by 66 young people, aged 10–25+. The majority fell within the 15–24 age group.

We then ran a one-off focus group with seven young people aged 12–19 who had all taken part in the programme. We divided the young people into two age groups, 11–13 and 14–18, to identify the different needs of young people with weight issues. They also explored potential solutions that could help to overcome barriers. The aims were to reflect on the findings from the research and to get young people's views on taking part in the research and implications for the future.

Involving specific marginalised groups of young people

Through the three projects outlined earlier, we involved a wide range of young people with different needs and experience. This section outlines how we were able to meet the specific needs of these groups of young people within each project.

'I find typing much easier than talking, and I know I'm not the only one – although of course everyone is different, so I think generally it's important to have some variety in communication options.' – *Webchat participant*

'I think the environment in A&E is difficult. It can be crowded with bright lights and noise. Often there is a lack of clear structure and this can be hard for individuals on the spectrum.' – *Webchat participant*

Involving autistic young people

We felt it was very important to hear the views of autistic young people when addressing acute care because of the particular issues they face when physically distressed or in high stress environments. As a neurological disorder that affects communication and makes people sensitive to stimulation, autism can make healthcare visits a particular challenge (CNN, 2016). We partnered with the specialist organisation Ambitious about Autism who recruited young people to take part in our Acute Care project. When the support worker contacted the young people, they decided that they felt much more comfortable having web discussion rather than a face-to-face meeting, and this kind of flexibility is critical in participation work. The group had an established forum that AYPH's Youth Participation Coordinator was invited to join on a temporary basis, and a two-hour time slot was organised in advance with the young people.

In this webchat, they discussed the particular barriers autistic young people face when accessing acute care services. They shared stories about sensory overload in Accident and Emergency and different experiences of pain being misunderstood or dismissed by health professionals (see Box 5.1). In response to these, the participants suggested a number of practical ideas about how acute care environments could be improved, some of which were based on positive experiences they had in a range of different healthcare settings. This willingness to be flexible and meet the young people in the environment where they felt most comfortable resulted in meaningful participation of many more young people than would have attended a traditional face-to-face focus group. For more on successfully involving autistic young people see case study 1 in Box 5.2.

Box 5.1: Response from survey respondent

'On one occasion, despite needing to be in A and E I ended up leaving due to sensory overload and ended up having to be sent back later in the day (and ended up be an inpatient in hospital, as my asthma was out of control). I also experience pain quite differently from other people which does not tend to be taken into account, even when I have explained this. On one occasion having injured my arm I ended up at the hospital. When they were examining my arm they didn't explain that they wanted me to say where it was painful and so I didn't volunteer any information about this as I didn't know that is what they needed to know. They told me off for wasting time as it seemed fine. However, one member of A and E staff decided it was worth x-raying just to make sure nothing was wrong which went on to show I had broken it and needed a cast etc. This experience though has made me more nervous about having to attend A and E in the future.'

Involving young people with HIV

Due to fears around stigma, young people growing up with HIV often choose not to or are discouraged from disclosing their condition to others (Hamblin, 2011; Hogwood et al, 2013; Grainger, 2016). Conversations with young people in the course of our participation work have revealed to us that although young people with HIV are frequent users of health services, they rarely get involved in general participation projects because they cannot share their experiences publicly. Our work with them has been predicated on the understanding that they will only participate through their specialist support service and not in open group activities. AYPH believed it was necessary to find a way of incorporating their views into our Acute Care project so we partnered with the CHIVA with whom we had an existing, positive working relationship. Although the young people were happy to attend a face-to-face workshop with the Youth Participation Coordinator, we knew from the beginning that it would not be possible for them to attend the larger group film-making workshop and maintain their anonymity. For this reason, we had to find an alternative way for their voices to be included in the final resource.

Knowing that not every young person would feel comfortable sharing personal stories in a group setting, we set up an anonymous survey where they could share any experience (good or bad) that they felt would provide important learning on acute care. Although the original project brief only required us to create a short film with the participants, we decided to also develop an infographic that highlighted some of the important messages we had collected through the workshops and anonymous survey. As a result, we were able to incorporate powerful quotes and messages from young people with HIV into a second resource that could be shared widely via social media.[1] Taking on this extra work was a necessary step to ensure that the voices of young people not often heard in any health context beyond HIV services were considered equally alongside other patient groups.

'There is a difference between empathy and sympathy. When people are sympathetic it's all well and good and nice to know that they care but they can't necessarily be on the same emotional level as me – unless you've had something similar happen to you, it's hard to empathise ... As a group we've become quite close-knitted and obviously we talk to each other a lot more now because we've got some similar experiences.'
– Health Advocate

Involving young people affected by sexual exploitation

Before AYPH's Be Healthy project (see earlier), group participation work in the field of CSE was very limited. Concerns about safeguarding, re-traumatising young people and anonymity around such a sensitive subject were effective barriers to developing group participation opportunities. As many CSE services are crisis-focused and primarily offer individual support, Be Healthy decided to offer financial support to partner projects in recognition of the extra staff time needed to involve young people in a participation project. Due to the shame and stigma surrounding CSE, facilitators developed and ran all activities using a third person lens, and there was never an expectation that participants would talk about their individual experiences. Trust was built up slowly and locally in small groups before bringing young people together from different projects and locations. Together we wrote and signed group agreements at each meeting so that everyone involved – including facilitators and support workers – understood their rights and responsibilities in group settings.

Be Healthy used creativity and storytelling to highlight needs of young people affected by CSE. Developing storyboards for an animated film allowed participants to incorporate important elements of their own stories without having to reveal their experiences to each other. Near the end of the project, some of the participants told us they felt prepared to tell more of their stories, so we supported each of them to write their own case studies which highlighted how the project affected them. These case studies gave them the opportunity to take back control of their stories, something they all felt had been removed from them by professionals when safeguarding procedures were triggered.

'In November, I was supported to give a presentation to a group of professionals. I never thought I'd be able to do that. It was nerve-wracking but it was worth it.' – *Health Advocate*

Before we asked participants to present their work publicly the facilitators ran an activity that helped the group define themselves collectively. This established exactly how they were comfortable presenting themselves as a group and how they wanted other people to talk about them. The participants chose to be known by their new active role of Be Healthy Health Advocates, moving away from the passive role of 'young people affected by CSE'. Although this self-definition was an important preventive step, we also worked with them on techniques for dealing with potentially intrusive and inappropriate questions that may be asked in public settings. The Health Advocates went on to present their work at several conferences around the UK and two international conferences. This final stage was possible because the long-term project continually supported them to feel less isolated, to assert their own boundaries and to believe that their opinions mattered on health issues beyond CSE. For more on involving young people affected by CSE, see case study 2 in Box 5.2.

Involving young people with weight issues

As with many other marginalised groups listed earlier, we anticipated that young people with weight issues might find it difficult to talk openly about their own health needs in a group setting. With limited resources available for the work, we planned a one-off face-to-face meeting with a small group of young people who had been involved in the aforementioned Promise study.

'It's not as simple as eating right and exercise. Eating is a very emotional issue and should be treated with respect and dignity.' – *Survey respondent*

'I used to be an obese child between the ages of 9 and 19, however, I lost 5 stone at 19. I never worried about weight then but the fear of getting fat is worse. I'm psychologically worse now as a healthy-looking young woman than I was before. I suffer with binge eating disorder but everyone just laughs it off as if I'm having a bad day as I'm slim.' – *Survey respondent*

We were also asked to provide reflections from a wider group of young people – those with and without experiences of weight issues. To do this we designed an online survey to collect responses from as many young people with different experiences as possible, and a total of 66 responded (see the earlier link). An important part of this survey was a free text box where participants could write anything they thought was important about the health of young people with weight issues. Their answers revealed a strong emphasis on self-esteem, mental health and how oppressive it can feel to be defined by their weight, both by peers and medical professionals. These issues were mirrored in the results of the activity we ran with the focus group.

Short-term interventions like this leave little room to build up trust and familiarity between group members. For this reason, we encouraged the seven young people taking part to think about the needs, barriers and potential support of a fictional young person with weight issues. One of the most important issues this project revealed was how divergent the needs of young people with weight issues were from the focus of many health professionals. The research focused solely on the effectiveness of different weight loss strategies but when given an opportunity to talk, young people emphasised the importance of how they felt over how they looked in both forums. This makes a clear case for why young people's views should always be included in research and service development, despite any barriers or difficulties.

Box 5.2: Case Studies 1 and 2

Case Study 1: Know Your Normal by Jack Welch

'Know Your Normal' originated from members of Ambitious about Autism's (AaA) myVoice project, which gives autistic young people aged 16–25 a platform to engage and volunteer across a wide range of activities (both digitally or in-person). AaA granted money from the myVoice funding to invest in a six-month youth-led campaign, with a subject chosen by volunteers. A meeting in October 2016 revealed that mental health was a high priority issue and one that many autistic young people were experiencing.

There were two resources that young people had the opportunity to shape: a research paper and a toolkit for young people. I opted for the former. Three young volunteers were invited to work alongside researchers at the Centre for Research in Autism and Education (CRAE) to co-produce the document from the beginning. This was vital to our successful collaboration, as we felt to be equal partners in shaping the objectives of this research. We also felt we were doing something that would benefit the wider autism community.

We reviewed the research paper right until its publication. We then went on to present and record our findings to diverse audiences, including academics and SEN professionals. It was very rewarding to share our messages with those who would benefit from this most.

In the wider Know Your Normal project, we were dealing with a sensitive subject area for many young people and some of those experiences might impact on us personally or act as a 'trigger'. In addition, autistic people require different and tailored levels of support to enable them to effectively participate. This might mean giving greater flexibility with the workload expected of them or alternative methods of communicating. Adult professionals need to be aware of what is right for each individual and allow them to participate at a level which they feel comfortable with.

There were ethical risks in relation to the research as it involved conducting individual interviews for an in-depth understanding of people's experiences of the mental health system. Volunteers with AaA had agreed to take part, which meant those of us leading on the research could not conduct interviews as we already had a connection to some of the participants. We agreed to stand aside from the actual interviews but did assist in reading transcripts which were from participants who had no role within AaA.

Many autistic young people tend to be isolated and not understood by their peers. By creating an environment where they are working with people who understand their life experiences and are treated as equal members of the team, they are capable of thriving and feeling part of a community. Know Your Normal was an example of a successful participation project where contributions came principally from autistic people themselves. Autistic people, like other marginalised groups who can be excluded when opportunities are not actively inclusive, are more than able to inform, lead and support projects of all kinds.

Case Study 2: Be Healthy by Kirsche Walker

I was involved in the Be Healthy project from 2010 to 2014. I was still at school and had only been referred to Safe and Sound Derby a few weeks prior to joining. I did not fully understand what the group was but I knew I wanted to be a part of something that took the focus away from just me and focused on young people more generally.

I quickly discovered that there were many young people from up and down the country and from different organisations, all of whom had either directly or indirectly been affected by exploitation. At the time I was only 15 years old, and meeting other young people who had similar experiences flicked a switch in me. I started to realise that my experiences were not isolated and also that they were not ok. Throughout the project I gained an in-depth knowledge about the lack of education and resistance to young people's participation within youth services. With the staff as mentors and other young people as peer supports, being part of this group helped me not only develop as a person but also to heal from previous traumas.

I still feel very lucky to have been able to work with the staff who facilitated the Be Healthy project. Working with AYPH and the University of Bedfordshire's International Centre contributed to who I am as a person and how I have grown and developed. They made sure that everyone in the group felt that they had a place. It was clear that we could contribute as much or as little as we felt and that there was not any pressure for any of us to attend every meeting or even stay involved if it became too difficult. It was particularly flexible, and I credit this as one of the main reasons so many of us stayed involved in such a long project.

There were challenges to being a part of the project – and I assume it was the same for the staff. Sometimes young people would not be able to attend the sessions so the group dynamics changed from meeting to meeting. Saying this we all had different strengths and engagement levels and it just worked! It worked so well. Some people would delegate, some people would take a lead on the more creative sides of things and some would take a lead on discussion and writing. Although some of the young people involved had to leave before the end of the project, they all contributed to how our project turned out and the resources we developed.

Personally, one of the huge difficulties for young people getting and staying involved in projects like this is that we become known for our past experiences. I found it extremely hard to talk about my experiences and deal with the attention that it brought me and the issue of sexual exploitation. I started off not really knowing what my role in the Be Healthy project would be or how I would be of use. By the end I knew that I wanted to dedicate myself to helping young people take control of their own futures and be able to shape and influence different aspects of their lives. It felt like both a burden and a blessing to understand from such a young age the route I wanted to take in my personal and professional life.

I understand that for many professionals, academics and even young people participation can seem daunting or impossible at times. It is of course necessary to highlight the potential risks, failures, re-traumatisation and 'barriers' before participation groups can even be set up. It is just as vital to recognise that many young people may end up viewing these groups as lifesavers and game changers. The experience for us to be involved in something bigger than our own trauma is invaluable. We are able to carry the amazing skills and thinking that we develop in these groups into our own lives and careers. Instead of allowing the risks to deter you from creating these safe spaces, groups and opportunities for young people, use them to fuel your energy to make it easier for future young people's participation projects.

Discussion

As highlighted earlier, it is important to find out about the specific needs of different marginalised groups – preferably directly from the young people – and make every effort to meet them whenever running a participation project. Their involvement is vital in order to hold services to account and ensure they are designed to meet all young people's health needs (WHO, 2017). In this section, we will share some more overarching messages AYPH has drawn from the wide range of participation projects we have run.

Partnership working

The first hurdle many projects encounter is recruitment of participants, and a common concern is that too narrow a range of young people respond to open participation calls. We have found that working in partnership with specialist organisations in the field is the best way to make contact with and involve marginalised groups of young people. The same local specialist organisations health professionals should be aware of and signposting young people to are potential partner organisations for engagement and participation work (Rigby and Starbuck, 2018). These organisations have already developed trusted relationships with young people and know how to support their involvement most effectively. It is important that these partnerships are as reciprocal as possible as specialist organisations are often small and stretched to capacity. Sharing funding bids or offering financial support for staff time demonstrates that you value their work and expertise. They will also be more likely to work with you again on future projects.

Remuneration for marginalised young people

Working relationships with marginalised young people should also be reciprocal. Health conditions and disabilities often result in serious financial burdens for young people and their families. Some young people may be on benefits or living without any financial support from parents or carers. It is important not to assume that a young person can pay for travel or food out of their own pocket and wait to be reimbursed. Instead pay for travel in advance and provide meals or refreshments at any activities you are running (INVOLVE, 2016). AYPH also rewards young people with vouchers at the end of projects to demonstrate our appreciation for their time and work. If in doubt, speak to your specialist partner organisations to find out what the best approach is for the young people you will be working with.

Using distancing techniques

Marginalised young people are often expected to repeat their traumatic stories and experiences to a number of professionals in order to access support. As the aim of participation projects is not generally therapeutic or to provide direct support, this should never be expected of young people in order to participate. AYPH clarifies from the beginning that we don't expect young people to talk about their personal experiences in group settings, and we often include this in our group agreements. We develop activities that depersonalise the issues we are exploring, for example asking young people to think about and discuss issues through fictional characters. Lived experiences will obviously come out in these discussions but they can be shared safely by participants when they apply them to a character.

Using creativity

Another way to achieve distance from personal experience is to use creative approaches (Foster, 2015; Kara, 2015). Storytelling, film-making and animation are all methods that can effectively highlight the issues experienced by group members without attributing them to any individual. This is particularly useful when working with young people who need to remain anonymous. In our experience young people have fun developing dramatic stories together that demonstrate all the things that can possibly go wrong for someone in a similar situation. Giving space to hyperbole and imagination can be an empowering way to acknowledge past harm and move towards finding solutions. We employ simple, low-tech creative techniques so that young people maintain control of the whole process rather than having to bring in outside experts. We also ensure young people have full control over the editing process.

Building up trusting relationships with young people over time

Participation of marginalised groups of young people should build gradually. Expecting high-level engagement or responsibility from the start can result in failure and young people disengaging altogether. Young people who face stigma for their conditions or experiences often feel isolated and ashamed and therefore need extra time and support to develop the confidence to give presentations or speak publicly. Some young people will never get to that point so there must be a variety of ways for participants to contribute to any resources. When young people feel a sense of ownership of the project outputs, they are more likely to feel confident talking about and sharing them.

Understanding the different perspectives and priorities of young people and the health system

Young people and health service providers may not always agree about what is best or indeed possible. Recognising that different perspectives exist as well as managing expectations and compromise are key elements of participation work and co-designing services with young people. Good engagement can tackle this. When projects are being commissioned, it is vital to clarify everything with the funders and the young people from the start. Vague topic areas that can be perceived in different ways, different expectations about the amount of work involved and different ideas of what participation actually means are a few of the ways in which conflicts arise. When they do, the role of the facilitating agency should be to act as a buffer between the participants and commissioners so young people are never made to feel as if their work is not good enough. Their other role is to advocate for the idea that listening to the concerns and hopes of young people is always a learning opportunity for the professionals who work with them.

Sometimes this divergence emerges simply because the lives of professionals and young people are very different. Put simply, a health professional who spends the majority of their time working in a clinical setting will see health within that context. A young person who spends most of their time in school, with family or in their community will see their health in relation to all aspects of their life and experience. After working through situations where the agendas of commissioners and young people turned out to be hard to align, AYPH developed a participation agreement to be signed before the start of any new project. It outlines exactly what we mean by terms like 'participation' and 'youth-led' and makes it clear that we will promote young people's work on our website exactly as they created it. There is often much learning behind the scenes of a project that exists outside of any outputs. For this reason, we also write our own project reports to capture this learning and create more constructive recommendations for professionals. The best way to avoid problems arising at the end of a project is to involve young people from the start in ways that support their specific needs.

Drawing out particular messages from diverse groups of young people

Although there will be shared concerns among young people, marginalised or excluded young people will also have particular personal perspectives that have developed from their unique situations. We cannot guess what these might be unless we talk to them. In this section we unpack some examples of this arising from AYPH's work.

Even when the topic of a project is clearly defined and relevant to the participants, it is possible the focus will shift in directions the facilitators never anticipated. This is the nature of genuinely youth-led work, where the shared needs and concerns of the group dictate the direction of the project (Coyne and Harder, 2011; Baker et al, 2014). The Be Healthy project provides an interesting example of this process.

As there had been so little group participation work prior to Be Healthy, it was difficult to predict what a group of young people affected by CSE would want to focus on when working together. Power imbalance in intimate relationships is a major factor of any sort of sexual violence but when we discussed this as a group, participants felt it was impossible to influence change since it was so personal. This made them feel relatively powerless. But as we worked through these issues, the young people began to identify that one relationship where they did have some power was as service users. The participants' mood shifted and they felt able to speak with authority about how they wanted to be treated – and how they didn't want to be treated – by the professionals who were supporting them. If we hadn't been responsive to the needs and feelings of the group and allowed these discussions to happen organically, we may never have reached this point.

Digital health records is another subject that exemplifies the wide range of opinions and concerns different groups of young people can have due to their particular situations. AYPH was commissioned to create a survey to collect young people's views about how medical information is currently shared and the creation of digital health records. Of the 30 young people who responded to our survey, 87 per cent were positive about the idea of having easier access to their own medical records. Gaining more control of their own care was seen as a positive outcome although 70 per cent were concerned about how long parents and carers would continue to have access to their records.

We felt it was vital to incorporate the voices of more marginalised young people who face stigma because of their health conditions and set up two focus groups to complement the survey results. In one focus group, young people with mental health issues highlighted fears about accessing their own medical files and 'becoming obsessive' about reading the details. In the second focus group, young people with HIV expressed concerns that something as seemingly harmless as a list of their prescriptions would be an immediate indicator of their HIV status to anyone looking at their records. These specific concerns, based on young people's unique lived experiences, may never have been considered when developing digital health records. The reason they were included was down to the extra effort AYPH made to involve them in the project.

Conclusion

Recent years have seen a very welcome emphasis on incorporating the views of young people into the development of health services. These opportunities to engage must be extended to young people who may be more marginalised from the mainstream, and who may find it harder to get their voices heard. Examples from three AYPH projects have illustrated some of the challenges that good participation can bring in more complex cases, but they also show how these can be overcome. The case studies demonstrate how beneficial it is to be part of a group where shared experiences are acknowledged and dealt with in a sensitive and supportive way. Seeking young people's views in this way is particularly important for those who face stigma, discrimination and barriers to accessing services.

Translating these examples into healthcare practice is challenging, and different groups of young people may bring different and unique challenges. However, these examples have shown that there are also some common lessons to be learned about how best to maximise the engagement opportunity, and to give young people a chance to be heard. It is possible to involve young people in the design and delivery of health services, and it is also possible to incorporate the experiences of marginalised young people. Key to good practice is flexibility and willingness to take the perspective of the young people. In practice this can mean being prepared to meet the young people in the environment where they feel most comfortable, and to ensure that staff have the appropriate training and support to undertake this kind of work. In some cases, this means working with third parties, specialist services or other partnerships with the voluntary sector, who can potentially provide ongoing support to participants after the participation work is complete. It also means being realistic about the time it may take to build trust and share experiences. Over recent years there has been much more willingness to invest in this kind of work, and to ensure that health services are designed in partnership with those who use them. Everyone benefits when it is done right.

Note

1 www.youngpeopleshealth.org.uk/wp-content/uploads/2017/05/acute-care-flow-chart.png

References

Baker, L., Hutton, C. and Balgobin, E. (2014) *Evaluation of right here: A young people's mental health initiative of the Paul Hamlyn and Mental Health Foundations.* London: Institute for Voluntary Action Research.

Barnardo's (2012) *Cutting them free: How is the UK progressing in protecting its children from sexual exploitation?* Barkingside: Barnardo's.

Berrick, J.D., Frasch, K. and Fox, A. (2000) Assessing children's experiences in out-of-home care: Methodological challenges and opportunities. *Social Work Research,* 24 (2), pp 119–27.

British Youth Council (2015) *Young people's political participation: Research, reflections and recommendation.* London: British Youth Council.

CNN (2016) *Helping patients with autism navigate the stressful ER.* Available from: https://edition.cnn.com/2016/02/29/health/autism-patient-care-er/index.html

Coyne, I. and Harder, M. (2011) Children's participation in decision-making: Balancing protection with shared decision-making using a situational perspective. *Journal of Child Health Care,* 15 (4), pp 312–19.

Crowley, A. (2015) Is anyone listening? The impact of children's participation on public policy. *International Journal of Children's Rights,* 23 (3), pp 602–21.

DCSF (Department for Children, Schools and Families) (2009) *Safeguarding children and young people from sexual exploitation.* London: DCSF.

Electoral Commission (2002) *Voter engagement and young people.* London: Electoral Commission.

Foster, V. (2015) *Collaborative Arts-based Research for Social Justice.* London: Routledge.

Grainger, C. (2016) Understanding disclosure behaviours in HIV-positive young people. *Journal of Infection Prevention,* 18 (1), pp 35–9.

Hagell, A. (2013) *AYPH Be Healthy Project Evaluation.* London: AYPH.

Hamblin, E. (2011) *Just normal young people; Supporting young people living with HIV in their transition to adulthood.* A report from the Children and Young People HIV Network. London: National Children's Bureau.

Heerman, W., White, R. and Barkin, S. (2015) Pediatrics perspectives: Advancing informed consent for vulnerable populations. *Pediatrics,* 135 (3), e562–4.

Hogwood, J., Campbell, T. and Butler, S. (2013) I wish I could tell you but I can't: Adolescents with perinatally acquired HIV and their dilemmas around self-disclosure. *Clinical Child Psychology and Psychiatry,* 18 (1), pp 44–60.

INVOLVE (2016) *Reward and recognition for children and young people involved in research – Things to consider.* Southampton: INVOLVE. Available from: www.invo.org.uk/wp-content/uploads/2016/05/CYP-reward-and-recognition-Final-April2016.pdf

Kara, H. (2015) *Creative Research Methods in the Social Sciences: A Practical Guide.* Bristol: Policy Press.

NHS Institute for Innovation and Improvement (2013) *The Patient Experience Book.* London: NHS Institute for Innovation and Improvement.

Rigby, E. and Starbuck, L. (2018) Public health for paediatricians: Engaging young people from marginalised groups. *Archives of Disease in Childhood: Education and Practice,* 103 (4), pp 207–10.

United Nations General Assembly (1989) *Convention on the Rights of the Child.* United Nations, Treaty Series, vol. 1577. New York: United Nations.

WHO (2017) *Global accelerated action for the health of adolescents (AA-HA!) Guidance to support country implementation.* Geneva: World Health Organization.

YMCA/NHS (2016) *I am whole: A report investigating the stigma faced by young people experiencing mental health difficulties.* London: National Council of YMCAs.

PART III

Collaborative research in NHS services

6

Listening to learn: enhancing children and young people's participation in a large UK Health Trust

Barry Percy-Smith, Sarah Kendal,
Joanne McAllister and Barry Williams

Introduction

Involving children and young people in NHS services has become an imperative for Hospital Trusts and given momentum by the Patient and Public Involvement (PPI) initiative and organisations such as National Institute for Health Research (NIHR) INVOLVE. An overriding concern with attempts to 'involve' children and young people in health settings has been on seeking their views or advice on matters defined by health professionals and researchers. Yet with a growing ethos towards shared decision-making, co-production, and developments to the theory and practice of children's participation (Banks et al, 2018; Tisdall, 2013; Percy-Smith, 2018), there is a shift towards more active approaches to children's participation in healthcare settings that recognise the importance of involving children and young people in all phases of the project cycle and in a wider range of contexts. This chapter draws on a collaborative action inquiry project with a UK NHS Hospital Trust to share the experience of developing meaningful and effective opportunities for involving children and young people across the Trust. Different strategies adopted, as well as some of the issues and challenges faced, will be discussed. In particular, the chapter will critically reflect on the significance of participation as patient experience and the challenges of integrating children's participation into organisational cultures and systems. Emphasis is placed on the need for creativity and flexibility in work with children, the critical role of adults as advocates and the importance of integrating a learning ethos into systems and practices across the Trust.

Developing the participation of children and young people in healthcare settings has been slower than in many other sectors such as schools and broader contexts of local governance in local authorities (ECORYS, 2015), in spite of the PPI initiative. Emphasis in involving children and young people has predominantly focused on seeking consultation and advice from children and young people, for example, through the gold standard of young people's research advisory groups (Nuffield Council on Bioethics, 2015; Caldwell and Jarrett, 2018). Children's participation in health settings is primarily about influencing the way in which hospital services are delivered, and in turn experienced, by children and young people.

Within this broader context two main foci for participation are discernible. One concerns what is referred to as 'individual participation' concerning children's involvement in decisions about their own care. This has resulted in development of scholarly and practice interest in shared decision-making in health care (see for example Alderson, 1993; 2007; Moore and Kirk, 2010; Coyne and Harder, 2011; Coyne et al, 2014; Vasey et al, 2016; Smith and Kendal, 2018). Studies such as these highlight the complexities involved in seeking a balance between children influencing decisions about their own care and treatment and the professional duty of nurses and clinicians to uphold duties of care by minimising risk and optimising outcomes. The power dynamic at play becomes a moral and political issue when children demonstrate a clear capacity to consent and is particularly an issue for older children and young people (Coyne et al, 2014). In turn, Smith and Kendal (2018) argue that shared decision-making between health professionals and parents/carers of a child with a long-term health condition may change over time according to the criticality of the issue at hand.

The second key focus for children's participation concerns how the needs, views and experiences of children and young people collectively as a generational group can influence health service practices and strategy more generally. This focus for participation is less concerned with immediate individual healthcare decisions and more about strategic decision-making and practice developments affecting the way health services are delivered. While approaches to participation in individual healthcare decisions are tied up with the ethics, identity and power of healthcare professionals, seeking the collective voice and participation of young people is dependent on structures and practices of learning and development and an overriding culture and commitment to children's participation (Kirby et al, 2003). The *Hear by Right* standards developed by Badham and Wade (2003) are one model[1] to support the development and embedding of participation in health services, highlighting the importance of bringing about changes to culture, leadership, systems, strategies and staff values. These interpretations of participation were all central in different ways in the Hospital Trust discussed in this case study example. In addition, as this paper highlights, large organisations such as Hospital Trusts can progress towards developing an enabling culture and environment for children's participation by simply getting children and young people on site and involved in activities.

Developing children's participation within an NHS Hospital Trust

Within the context of imperatives to involve children more actively in evaluating and improving services within the Trust, initial steps had been taken through, for example, introducing patient feedback boxes on site. Yet as one member of staff stated, "It's all very well people coming to us with comments or queries, but if we never change anything as a result, it's just an administrative exercise." This concern captures one of the key challenges of enhancing children's participation: concerning how to ensure participation is not tokenistic but is a meaningful, effective and sustainable process (Sinclair, 2004) of enabling children to contribute to change. There is now widespread acknowledgement that children's participation involves more than simply having a say (Nolas, 2015), and instead involves more active roles in all phases of the decision-making or project cycle. In addition, as Percy-Smith (2010) and others (see for example Lundy, 2007; Tisdall, 2013) argue, how people listen, learn and respond to the contribution of children is also part of the participatory process (see also Kirby et al, 2003).

The Trust, in this case, similarly identified the central aim of 'ensuring children and young people's participation is integral to service evaluation and improvement'. What this implicitly meant was that the development of children and young people's participation in the Trust should be a comprehensive initiative across all parts of the Trust and involving all members of staff. This was reflected in the title and objectives for a children's participation project called 'Listening to Learn':

- to map where we are and what we have achieved with children's participation;
- to identify gaps and areas of development;
- to develop an infrastructure to improve children and young people's experiences of our services;
- to develop an organisational culture and system for involving children and young people beyond just hearing their views;
- to integrate children and young people's participation across the Trust and at all levels of decision-making.

Academic researchers worked on this project alongside Trust staff to inform and support ongoing developments through an active process of learning in action – reflecting on practice and identifying realistic possibilities for expanding children's participation. To achieve this the project adopted a collaborative action inquiry approach, which is essentially a participatory, experiential learning process to inform developments and build individual and collective capacity through engaged praxis of action and reflection. The idea behind such a participative action research process is to support staff as co-researchers in a process of critical inquiry with a view to researching and bringing about change (Weil, 1998; McTaggart et al, 2017) in the context of their own lives through iterative cycles of reflection, learning and action. Research in this case involves critically reflective inquiry into their own practice and systems as a form of practice-based research or, as Whitehead (2018) conceives such a process: through participation in developing 'living theories of action'. Carr and Kemmis (1986, p 162) state that: 'Action research is simply a form of self-reflective inquiry undertaken by participants in social situations in order to improve […] their own practices and realities, their understanding of these practices and the situations in which the practices are carried out'.

The intentions in this study were to facilitate staff in a developmental process to gain a better understanding of the state of play with respect to participation in the Trust, to reflect on and develop understanding of what participation might involve in the context of the Trust and from that, develop an action plan for what they felt needed to be done to develop an effective children's participation system. This was to be followed up by support in practice for different groups in implementing measures put in place, and through evaluating these measures, to then communicate successes to other parts of the Trust to support a process of whole system change.

The original design of the process was to have an initial workshop with key staff to capture good practice thus far, consider wider perspectives on theories and practices of children's participation and use this to identify where and how developments to practice could be made. The second stage was to work with children and young people to understand better their perspectives as service users to inform where changes to practice could be made. Changes would then be implemented and evaluated and then principles for good practice communicated more widely across the Trust supported by the production of a children's participation guide. In reality, events took their own course, the project team responding to other initiatives and priorities in the Trust that emerged and opportunities that presented themselves through partnership work with schools and the initiative of the volunteer coordinator. Workshops, interviews and consultations were still undertaken with staff and children, which in turn gave rise to action and developments, but happened in a more dynamic, emergent and serendipitous way.

Action research under different guises (such as the collaborative action inquiry approach adopted here) as a dynamic participative, action-focused learning approach is ideally suited to supporting inquiry and development of children's participation as it enables participants to be actively involved rather than recipients of a new edict. At the same time, initiatives of this kind are not neat and tidy and formulaic, rather are messy and complex within a context of multiple agenda, priorities and levels of commitment. Being responsive and emergent according to wider events and developments is key. Accordingly, in working with the Trust on this project we encountered numerous issues and challenges that influenced how the plan unfolded. In action research, difficulties encountered in the form of messiness, resistance and obstacles are part of the process of learning, and developing new ways of working and should not be edited out. In the following section we discuss some of the key issues and challenges we encountered.

Issues and challenges

In a recent evaluation of children's participation across the EU (ECORYS, 2015) a key finding was that while legislation existed across many public sectors to support children's participation, there was a problem for professionals understanding what this meant in practice. In this case study, we similarly found that practitioners, at best, struggled to understand how to realise participation in practice and, at worst, had a very limited understanding of, and commitment to, children's participation at all as reflected in one response from a participation lead: "There are real challenges with embracing patient voice, it is a constant struggle ... they say 'can't you do it?'" (Patient experience lead). While it is important to have participation champions such as a patient experience lead, developing a whole organisational culture of participation has to involve everyone. Challenging and changing the attitudes and values of staff may be key to developing a culture of participation, and especially difficult for staff who do not necessarily share a vision for children's participation. Moreover, there were a significant number of staff who felt that doing a good job was sufficient for their role and were apparently resistant to changing how they work to integrate children's participation. For example, some paediatric nurses argued that they are already providing child-centred care and struggled to see why and how they would provide more of a say to children and integrate participation into their role with many seeing participation as another thing to have to do in addition to an already time pressured working life. The wider context here is the challenge of seeking innovation with staff who are already feeling beleaguered.

Participation is so often still seen in terms of just hearing the voice of children. While this is of course important, effective participation involves more than just hearing children's views. There is now widespread acknowledgement that participation also involves being treated respectfully and being kept informed, having opportunities to talk things through and know what is happening, to exercise choice in terms of their own care, and to feel ok to voice concerns and anxieties (Nuffield Council on Bioethics, 2015). These issues are about participation as relational practice and involve practitioners working in more open, reflexive child-centred ways that value the creativity and contribution children can provide as partners in, rather than recipients of, care.

Hospital Trusts are large organisations with multiple strategic agendas playing out simultaneously, placing demands on different staff at different times. While Hospital Trusts readily express commitment to PPI, the way in which this necessarily manifests is in terms of enhancing effectiveness in healthcare provision tied to outcomes. In busy service delivery contexts, practice is invariably quite instrumental – meeting immediate clinical need, rather than being pre-occupied with children's concerns which might be seen as more peripheral such as whether the waiting room feels like a welcoming environment. Yet, evidence suggests that through involving children more effectively, services are better able to improve outcomes for patient benefit (Kirby, 2004). In this case study Hospital Trust, while there was support for this participation initiative at a strategic level, there was a lack of active buy-in at a middle management level. In reality the children's participation agenda was progressed by a small number of individuals through a series of activities and 'actions for change'.

Actions for change to enhance the participation of children

In our 'Learning to Listen' workshop, we used a cooperative inquiry process to understand better the challenges affecting children and young people's participation. Staff who attended engaged in a subsequent cycle of action inquiry to explore where they felt action needed to be focused to develop participation. The popular metaphor of the tree bearing fruits of change was used with easy pickings (things that could be actioned easily) at the bottom and measures that take more time at the top. What was interesting was the extent to which staff identified *'communicating and relating to children and young people'* as key in addition to ensuring the necessary systemic arrangements to support both staff and children. In contrast to common approaches to involving children that focus on the quality of environment of the waiting rooms such as the colour of the walls and providing a companion for the lonely goldfish in the fish tank, as much as these are important, we document a broader set of actions that reflect a more elaborate and far-reaching understanding of children and young people's participation in healthcare settings. We discuss these actions according to three areas of activity:

Information and outreach: making connections

In many cases children do not have experience of a hospital environment until they need to use it. As a result, children often exhibit anxiety about what will happen when they do need to go into hospital. A key focus for action was in providing information and raising awareness of children and young people about what it is like to be in hospital and what hospital staff do. While availability of information is not in itself a form of participation, it is nonetheless an important precursor affecting participation and, as this case illustrates, linked closely to patient experience. Raising awareness was achieved in a number of ways.

First, through outreach into schools to talk about what hospitals do, but also for children to have an opportunity to ask questions. This follows an ethos of **corporate citizenship** laying the foundations for more (pro)active engagement by talking about what the NHS does and how children and young people can be involved. In so doing, children not only benefit from learning about their health service, but this may also provide a form of careers education as some children may develop an interest in pursuing a career as a nurse or clinician. In this project, school visits were linked to recruitment of volunteers to take on more active roles in the Hospital Trust (see following section). Connections with some local schools were already in place, but were built on in the course of this work involving bringing children into the hospital to take part in a research workshop ('Getting it right for children & young people') to capture the experiences and views of children to inform hospital practice.

The second way of raising awareness in a fun way was through visits and 'takeover days' in which groups of children and young people come into the hospital and get to see first-hand different areas of the hospital's activities. Takeover days are a common approach wherein children come into the hospital for a day and look behind the scenes, speak to patients and staff and comment on the hospital environment and how they think it might impact on children and young people. Ideas and improvements from children and young people have included having name boards beside their bed to encourage staff to engage in a more personal way and having a hospital radio station. Some children from a local primary school talked to us about what they would like to hear on the radio if they were in hospital; following negotiations, we were able to facilitate a school-based activity in which they planned a two-hour hospital radio slot, which they subsequently delivered.

Developing partnership work with schools is an important element of public involvement and at the same time, for schools, develops educational experiences beyond the classroom in wider community settings (Bentley, 1998). It is widely acknowledged that it is good practice and often essential to build a relationship with participants before working with them (Kirby, 2004). This is also the case with children and participation. Expecting children and young people to step forward and 'participate' is unrealistic if there is no context. However, by going into schools and talking with young people, hearing their perspectives and sharing information about the work of hospitals, provides an 'opening' that can lead to opportunities for children and young people's participation (Shier, 2001). Through the partnerships developed with schools, dialogues with children are opened up providing education and awareness raising for children about illness, healing and hospitals, while at the same time providing insights into how children see hospitals and hospital staff.

Active engagement of children and young people

By its very nature participation is about active engagement. Participation is so often understood as just being about hearing the views of young people that adult professionals can then take on board in what they do, often reflected in the oft-used mantra "we asked, you said, we did". Yet, as well intentioned as this sounds, limiting children's participation in this way denies opportunities for children to participate in more active and direct ways, for example through volunteering initiatives, that can provide valuable inputs into learning and improvement initiatives in hospitals. In this project, children and young people were actively engaged in a range of ways that sought to harness their expertise and perspectives for specific purposes.

The first form of active participation involved a classic example of **co-design with children and young people** and concerned involving children in helping the hospital develop a maternal bereavement suite. This is not just about valuing children's input to the design of such an environment, but also provides valuable opportunities for children to learn and talk about death, bereavement, miscarriages and so on. In this particular case children raised the money themselves for the artwork by putting on events. In doing so, the children developed skills and confidence as well as a culture of active citizenship.

Often children's participation is seen in terms of inputting into an adult-led initiative that adults then implement. Yet there is now mounting evidence that demonstrates the ways in which young people can participate directly through taking on **active**

roles in providing support and services themselves. Three noteworthy examples of children providing support and services emerged in the course of this work. The first set of initiatives concerned young people taking active roles in providing services through reading to patients with dementia and involving college students in providing hairdressing services for these patients. In contrast to the conventional 'voice in decision-making' focus in children's participation, these two examples provide excellent illustrations of how children and young people can participate as fellow citizens and members of a community through interpersonal interactions. In the case of the reading initiative, this provided educational benefits for the young people by providing reading practice, learning about dementia, as well as developing confidence. At the same time patients benefited from having someone inputting into their experience in non-medical ways to contribute to a more humanising hospital experience. In the second example, college students have the opportunity to gain experience as trainee hairdressers, while patients benefit by feeling better having their hair done. Perhaps more importantly here is a deeper value of human connection and the benefits of inter-generational interaction reflected in the delight, smiling faces and positive feedback from patients whose experience was enriched. One of the ideas for action that emerged from this work was to harness young people's experiences as **'expert patients' providing peer-to-peer support**, for example having young people to support other young people when they come into hospital.

A variation of takeover days is where children come into the hospital to inspect different areas of the hospital and provide ideas about, for example, how to make hospital environments or practices more child-friendly. **Inspections** are a worthwhile way of children sharing their views about hospital environment and practices, while simultaneously providing an opportunity for children to become more familiar with hospital environments in case they need to use them. Inspections can produce issues through the lens of children's perspectives that can be used to challenge hospital staff to make changes in ways that are more closely aligned to children's needs, perspectives and experiences. In this Hospital Trust, a '15-step challenge' was established in which young people identified changes they felt were needed from their perspective. This involved children identifying things that they think are important for keeping children safe and improving their experience. Many are relatively simple, no-cost options such as staff remembering to smile and ensuring the time to listen to children's concerns.

Seeking ideas and perspectives from children is perhaps the simplest form of children's participation and, while not sufficient in itself in realising the wider possibilities of children's participation, is nonetheless important in ensuring hospital practices are geared most effectively in response to the needs of different children. In one of the project workshops children from local schools were brought into the hospital to share their views and experiences about a range of issues pertinent to the development of children and young people's participation and child-friendly practice. An important issue in developing effective participation with children and young people that emerged from the project workshop inquiry with staff concerned '*effective communication*'. This requires staff having the necessary skills and qualities to engage with children such as an awareness of the importance of giving time for the child to talk, share their concerns and ask questions, empathy, non-verbal communication and so on. One of the initiatives undertaken involved children with communication difficulties training staff to understand their communication needs[2] and the use of non-verbal communication skills including signing. The enthusiasm and skills of the children encouraged staff present to learn signing, and this has now developed into a certified training provision with children's input.

It is now quite common for children and young people to be involved in **recruitment** processes, and in this project children provided some important perspectives for person specifications for recruiting new NHS hospital staff members and ideas for interview questions. These included posing scenarios about how they would engage with a child with a serious illness, how they would comfort a child before life-threatening surgery or what they would do if they made a mistake. What was interesting was that most of children's issues reflected concerns about seeking reassurance if they were a patient.

However, staff said there was not the time to involve children in interviewing even though parents were involved. To overcome this, the matter was taken to HR to amend policy so that people have to involve children.

Systematising and sustaining children and young people's participation

What is evident from these examples is the extent to which children and young people can participate in a broader set of ways than simply expressing a view to adults to inform decisions and services provided. These may be considered as forms of 'social' participation of children and young people based on asset-based approaches in which children's contributions are valued as equal citizens. While these are an important part of the mosaic of children's participation, opportunities for children and young people to influence policy and practice development are equally important. We have highlighted ways in which children and young people can be involved in service evaluation through inspections and in recruitment. However, developing ways in which children and young people can participate meaningfully, effectively and sustainably (Sinclair, 2004) in key decision-making is harder to achieve. As other papers in this volume highlight, for young people to contribute to strategic decision-making depends on provision of structures and opportunities for dialogue, learning and collaborative decision-making that collectively are key elements of what is now commonly referred to as **co-production**.

In initiatives such as this project to enhance children's participation, there can sometimes be a desire to 'get the strategy right' before doing anything. Getting started with a few activities can be beneficial in creating a sense of momentum through achieving quick wins and developing partnerships and connections with children and young people. Indeed, making things happen is arguably what is most important rather than focusing on getting a strategy. At the same time, in spite of the positive energy and impact from the different participation initiatives put in place, they were not joined up in a coherent way, making it difficult to systematise and sustain through organisational change. While staff can take the initiative and make things happen, as was the case to a significant extent in this work, developing a culture of participation is more effective when it is **integrated with and supported by management and systems** (Badham and Wade, 2003; Percy-Smith, 2010). This involves not only actively embracing forms of participation but paying attention to the **systems and practices that need to be put in place** to reflect, support and facilitate changes and developments in practice and make participation happen as a matter of course rather than a one-off event.

In this initiative a number of practice development measures were identified. First, as mentioned earlier, **communication and quality of professional relationships** were noted as being key to effective participation. This primarily concerns participation in individual care encounters, for example, children saying that doctors and nurses should regularly communicate with children throughout their hospital care experience, however long or short, to ensure they have an opportunity to say how they feel at different stages. This requires in-service training to ensure staff acknowledge the importance of how they inter-relate with children and young people and develop their skills accordingly. Effective and personable professional-child relationships are key to the child's patient experience and need to encompass asset-based perspectives with respect to children's participation.

Second, the Learning to Listen project workshop with staff uncovered the centrality of staff **working practices** that affect a more comprehensive uptake of, and proactive support for, children's participation practices. These included the challenge of conflicting demands, time constraints, declining staff numbers, insufficiently working as a team and feeling a sense of excitement and joy in their work rather than feeling frustrated and that they are always battling against something. Children's participation therefore needs to involve ensuring staff are also empowered and supported by having the necessary resources, capacity and systems to enable children's participation. This needs also to involve an organisational culture of child participation in which involvement is integrated as a norm rather than an exception as well as the creation of a positive working environment that enables and values staff views and expertise. In spite of most staff acknowledging the value of child-friendly processes, some also readily suggested that children's participation should be undertaken by someone else. So often staff feel undervalued and feel they too do not have a voice and influence in the system, even though they have significant insight into key issues and challenges in practice. Developing a culture of participation involves ensuring there are systems for practice-based learning and reflection within which the views and experiences of staff are also valued.

Third, while it has been noted that a range of activities and opportunities are important for engaging young people, there is a danger that these become another thing to do. Joining up multiple agenda appears to be a sensible strategy within a sector with multiple bottom lines. In this project children's participation was framed structurally by a **Children and Young People's Patient Experience Group** (CYPPEG) integrating it into wider hospital evaluation and governance processes. This appears prudent in that developments are tied to patient outcomes, yet at the same time there is a danger that children's participation and the experience of 'children as patients' becomes conflated and the meanings and values lost.

Fourth, while different types of patient feedback (for example end-of-care evaluation forms, suggestion boxes and so on) are commonly used, frequently there is an absence of systems to process and **learn from feedback and integrate into service improvement processes** in a systematic way. In a pressurised and resource-scarce NHS, diverting staff resources to processing patient feedback may not be seen as a priority, yet this could be easily undertaken by volunteers supervised by admin personnel and overseen by the head of patient engagement together with Children and Young People's Patient experience groups.

Reflections

Considerable progress has been made in this Hospital Trust in engaging children and young people, and to a greater extent this is down to the hard work and dedication of a small number of staff for whom children's participation falls within their brief. The experience in this Trust is also refreshing in that the focus wasn't solely on reproducing customary project-based opportunities for involving children through, for example, young people's advisory groups or one-off consultations, and instead focused on developing a wider spectrum of opportunities for participation in more direct and active ways in order to develop and sustain involvement. However, while there is an undeniable rationale for the developments that have happened, these have to a large extent concerned the low-hanging fruit, the safer issues for children to be involved in. There has been less progress in changing the culture of hospital nursing staff in developing children's involvement at an individual level in their care planning and at a collective level, having structures, systems and practices for integrating children and young people's views and experiences into strategic decisions making and using learning from that to inform change. Indeed, interviews with Trust staff suggest that in spite of the value of the engagement initiatives with children and young people that have happened, there was little evidence of children having significant influence in challenging structures and processes in the Trust and with little sense that this was either feasible or desirable.

At the same time, Trust representatives continue to state that: 'Children and young people's participation should be part of everything we do.' Providing the necessary education and awareness to inform how children and young people's participation is developed is often best achieved experientially by just simply starting to make things happen through activities and initiatives that can begin to set a precedence and momentum for change. In short, placing emphasis on action and learning from that. However, time continues to be an issue for many staff:

> 'I feel that the main issue regarding participation of children and young people is time and lack of staff. Most of my colleagues do participation as much as they can within time constraints. The NHS's problems are the same as always – not enough time.'

Although there is support at a strategic level, day-to-day pressures were identified by staff as being likely to dominate people's priorities unless there was a clear push from champions in the form of individuals people could relate to. Yet, for children's participation to be truly reflected across the Trust there remains a challenge in getting this more clearly embedded in Trust policy and practice, rather than just as a part of the quality improvement agenda, backed by resources and linked to outcome measures.

Notes

[1] See also Anne Crowley's standard developed in Wales (Crowley and Skeels 2010).
[2] See also Roulstone and McLeod (2011).

References

Alderson, P. (1993) *Children's Consent to Surgery*. Milton Keynes: Open University Press.

Alderson, P. (2007) Competent children? Minors' consent to health care treatment and research. *Social Science and Medicine*, 65 (11), pp 2272–83.

Badham, B. and Wade, H. (2003) *Hear by Right: Standards for the Active Involvement of Children and Young People*. Leicester: National Youth Agency.

Banks, S., Hart, A., Pahl, K. and Ward, P. (eds) (2018) *Co-producing Research: A Community Development Approach*. Bristol: Policy Press.

Bentley, T. (1998) *Learning Beyond the Classroom: Education for a Changing World*. London: Routledge.

Caldwell, P. and Jarrett, C. (2018) In their own words: Engaging young people in a youth research advisory group: Letters to the editor. *Journal of Paediatrics and Child Health*, 54 (1), pp 107–8.

Carr, W. and Kemmis, S. (1986) *Becoming Critical: Education, Knowledge and Action Research*. London: Routledge Falmer.

Coyne, I. and Harder, M. (2011) Children's participation in decision-making: Balancing protection with shared decision-making using a situational perspective. *Journal of Child Health Care*, 15 (4), pp 312–19.

Coyne, I., Amory, A., Kiernan, G. and Gibson, F. (2014) Children's participation in shared decision-making: Children, adolescents, parents and healthcare professionals' perspectives and experiences. *European Journal of Oncology Nursing*, 18 (3), pp 273–80. [Last accessed: 21st August 2018 from: https://doi.org/10.1016/j.ejon.2014.01.006]

Crowley, A. and Skeels, A. (2010) Getting the measure of children and young people's participation: an exploration of practice in Wales, in B. Percy-Smith, and N. Thomas (eds.) *A Handbook of Children and Young People's Participation: Perspectives from Theory and Practice*, London: Routledge.

ECORYS (2015) *Evaluation of legislation, policy and practice on children's participation in the European Union.* EU DG Justice.

Kirby, P. (2004) *A guide to actively involving young people in research: For researchers, research commissioners and managers.* Brighton: PK Consulting/INVOLVE.

Kirby, P., Lanyon, C., Cronin, K. and Sinclair, R. (2003) *Building a culture of participation: Involving children and young people in policy, service planning, delivery and evaluation.* (Report and Handbook) London: DfES.

Lundy, L. (2007) 'Voice' is not enough: Conceptualising Article 12 of the United Nations Convention on the Rights of the Child. *British Educational Research Journal*, 33 (6), pp 927–42.

McTaggart, R., Nixon, R. and Kemmis, S. (2017) Critical participatory action research. In L. Rowell, C. Bruce, J.M. Shosh and M. Riel (eds.) *The Palgrave International Handbook for Action Research.* New York: Palgrave Macmillan, pp 21–35.

Moore, L. and Kirk, S. (2010) A literature review of children's and young people's participation in decisions relating to health care: Children's and young people's participation in decisions. *Journal of Clinical Nursing*, 19 (15–16), pp 2215–25.

Nolas, S.-M. (2015) Children's participation, childhood publics and social change: A review. *Children & Society*, 29 (2), pp 157–67.

Nuffield Council on Bioethics (2015) *Children and clinical research: Ethical issues.* Available from: http://nuffieldbioethics.org/wp-content/uploads/Children-and-clinical-research-full-report.pdf

Percy-Smith, B. (2010) Councils, consultation and community: Rethinking the spaces for children and young people's participation, *Children's Geographies*, 8 (2), pp 107–22. 10.1080/14733281003691368

Percy-Smith, B. (2018) Participation as learning for change in everyday spaces. In C. Baraldi and T. Cockburn (eds.) *Theorising Childhood: Citizenship, Rights and Participation*, Palgrave MacMillan, pp 159–86.

Roulstone, S. and McLeod, S. (eds.) (2011) *Listening to Children and Young People with Speech Language and Communication Needs*, Albury, Nr Guildford: J&R Press.

Shier, H. (2001) Pathways to participation: Openings, opportunities and obligations. *Children & Society*, 15 (2), pp 107–17.

Sinclair, R. (2004) Participation in practice: Making it meaningful, effective and sustainable. *Children & Society*, 18 (2), pp 106–18.

Smith, J. and Kendal, S. (2018) Parents' and health professionals' views of collaboration in the management of childhood long-term conditions. *Journal of Pediatric Nursing*, 43, pp 36–44.

Tisdall, E.K.M. (2013) The transformation of participation? Exploring the potential of 'transformative participation' for theory and practice around children and young people's participation. *Global Studies of Childhood*, 3 (2), pp 183–93.

Vasey, J., Smith, J., Kirschbaum, M. and Chirema, K. (2016) G327(P) tokenism or true partnership: Parental involvement in the child's acute pain care. *Archives of Disease in Childhood*, 101, A189.

Weil, S. (1998) Rhetorics and realities in public service organisations: systemic practice and organisational as Critically Reflexive Action Research (CRAR). *Systemic Practice and Action Research* 11: 37–61.

Whitehead, J. (2018) *Living Theory Research as a Way of Life*, Bath: Brown Dog Books & The Self Publishing Partnership.

7

Shifting sands: trying to embed participation in a climate of change

Louca-Mai Brady, Emily Roberts,
Felicity Hathway and Lizzy Horn

Introduction

The Community Children's Health Partnership (CCHP) was, at the time of the research project discussed in this chapter, a partnership between North Bristol National Health Service Trust (the NHS Trust) and the children's charity Barnardo's. Working in close collaboration in service design, delivery and evaluation, the ambition was to provide equitable and integrated care with a focus on participation and the voices of children and young people (CYP) from the outset. Along with the health services provided by the NHS Trust CCHP included a dedicated participation service called HYPE (Helping Young People to Engage) delivered by Barnardo's.

The CCHP was a case study for Louca–Mai's doctoral research on 'embedding children and young people's participation in health services and research' (Brady, 2017). The authors were involved in an action research project which sought to develop and embed participation across all CCHP services and identify learning to inform the development of CYP's participation in the development and delivery of health services. At the time

Emily was the Barnardo's Participation Manager and had been involved as a key partner in the CCHP from the outset, and Felicity and Lizzy were involved through the HYPE project as young advisors. The project involved health professionals, young people and Barnardo's participation service working collaboratively to develop a strategy and framework to support children's participation in the organisation.

This chapter starts by outlining the background and methods used in the project, before exploring the lessons from this project for the involvement of CYP in health policy and services from both professional and young people's perspectives. We also consider events which took place after the completion of the project, when the CCHP was recommissioned and restructured, highlighting the risks of competitive tendering and NHS commissioning processes on the embedding of CYP's participation in health services. This chapter also draws on a previous publication by the authors (Brady et al, 2018).

The CCHP participation story

The CCHP was a partnership between the NHS Trust and Barnardo's, contracted from 2009 to 2016 to deliver children's community health services in Bristol and South Gloucestershire. It employed over 800 staff in mental and physical health services including CAMHS (Child and Adolescent Mental Health Services), health visiting, school nursing, physiotherapy, speech and language therapy, occupational therapy, community paediatricians and seven specialist services, including an inpatient adolescent unit. The ambition was to provide cohesive, equitable and integrated care with a focus on participation and the voice of the child:

> Service user participation is an important part of our service and we are keen to involve children and young people to help us improve the services we offer. (CCHP, 2014a)

Within the services which came together to form the CCHP there had been pockets of interest in participation, for example a service user participation group in the CAMHS services. But in an e-mail sent to Louca-Mai during the project Emily said she felt that this:

> ...wasn't backed up by serious management support so [participation had] tended to focus on getting things like water available in the waiting room and magazines [rather than getting CYP's input in service design, delivery and policy]. There was a growing interest [in participation] but without any structure. Many services had never evaluated their work or thought to ask families or children about what they thought. In disability services they had historically had parents come to talk at their away days but it was hard to know what to do with the feedback they were given. Most CCHP services had [also] never been tendered before. (Roberts, 2016)

Barnardo's, a national voluntary sector organisation with an established culture of participation, were subcontracted by the NHS Trust to support and drive service user participation within CCHP services. The Barnardo's element of CCHP was called HYPE: Helping Young People (and children and families) Engage and aimed to:

> support children and families to have a say, recognising them as experts in their own lives so they can influence how their health services are delivered. HYPE works with both health workers and managers to support the involvement of children and young people. (CCHP, 2015a)

The CCHP core stated values were and remain: 'respect for the unique worth of each child and young person, outcome-focused and innovative, child and young person at the centre, accessible and equitable services [and] service user participation at all levels' (CCHP, 2014b). The related charter, created by young people, says that CYP using CCHP services should:

- have a choice of how information is presented and it should be easy to understand and age appropriate;
- have a right to be treated as individuals and to not be patronised or judged;
- have a right to be seen by health workers who are welcoming, patient and understanding;
- be given the opportunity to change their health worker and where possible be given a choice of male or female worker;
- have a say in what information is shared and with whom;
- have a say in arranging their appointments, in places which are clean, comfortable and accessible. (CCHP, 2016a)

During our project a Care Quality Commission (CQC) inspection rated the CCHP as Outstanding and found that:

> *Involving children and young people was routinely undertaken across the CCHP and was seen as an example of outstanding service nationally* ... partnership working was routinely included in every aspect of their work. The sole purpose of the CCHP was to improve services for children and young people. (CQC, 2015, p 4, emphasis added)

The CQC report goes on to say:

> User participation was routinely undertaken. Benefits had been demonstrated such as effective communication, relationship building, active listening and had improved [CYP's] ... and their parents' or carer's wellbeing.
>
> The HYPE project was run by Barnardo's project workers and aligned to the two local authority areas in Bristol and South Gloucestershire as part of the CCHP. This partnership was unique and was being observed by senior researchers, government

and health organisations across the country. The partnership was about bringing together the skills and experience of Barnardo's and North Bristol NHS Trust to address inequalities in health provision to improve outcomes for all children and young people and their families, especially the most vulnerable, and to have children's experience at the centre of decision making.

A unique example of participation was the inclusion of young people on interview panels. Young people were given mentoring and preparation training. Monitoring that had been done following interviews showed that 100% of both professionals and young people felt the young people had significant influence in the final decision for recruitment of new staff. (CQC, 2015, p 6)

But while there was a commitment to give CYP's views and experiences a stronger platform in CCHP, this was a challenge to a hierarchical healthcare culture where the power to make decisions is held by professionals as experts. At the time this project started there was a cohort of engaged and active CYP and families, and an increasing number of professionals and services with an interest in developing participation practice. The relationship between the Barnardo's service and CCHP staff was cementing in pockets but was still fragile at other points, and CCHP were looking for ways to improve and consolidate practice so that CYP's participation would be understood and owned by staff and CYP across the organisation.

Embedding participation: the CCHP as a case study

The partnership was attempting to put into practice many of the ideas Louca-Mai wanted to explore about what it meant to embed CYP's participation in healthcare practice and look in more depth at what happens between rhetoric and reality. Following agreement with senior CCHP managers the CCHP became a case study for Louca-Mai's doctoral research on 'embedding children and young people's participation in health services and research', undertaken as part of a studentship funded by the University of the West of England as part of a programme of research led by Professor Barry Percy-Smith (Brady, 2017). CCHP were identified as providing a unique opportunity to explore what it means to embed CYP's participation in health services given the organisation's commitment to CYP's participation from the outset, as well as the multi-disciplinary and multi-agency nature of the organisation. Facilitated by support from senior leadership in the NHS Trust and Barnardo's, Louca-Mai worked with CCHP managers and staff, young people and other stakeholders through a series of collaborative action research workshops between September 2013 and June 2015.

Approach and methods

The overall research project used an action research approach to understand how organisational culture, systems and practice support or create barriers to young people's participation, and to locate this within a framework of participatory, rights-based research (Beazley and Ennew, 2006). Action research is a way of 'working towards practical outcomes, and also creating new forms of understanding' (Reason and Bradbury, 2008, p 2), in a process of critical inquiry with a wider group of stakeholders 'including policy makers and those "on the receiving end" of policy' (Torrance, 2011, p 577).

A core group of CCHP professionals and young people were involved throughout the process ('active partners' in Box 7.1) along with others who were involved at different stages.

Box 7.1: Research participants

- NHS Trust and voluntary sector organisation managers and commissioners (active partners);
- staff in a range of services across the Health Partnership (active partners);
- young people involved in CCHP participation activity (active partners);
- CCHP management groups (focus group participants);

- members of a learning disability service's parents group (focus group participants);
- members of the Clinical Commissioning Group (focus group participants);
- organisations collaborating with the Health Partnership and other stakeholders (focus group and interview participants).

Brady, 2017

The action research process typically involves self-reflective cycles of planning a change, acting and observing the process and consequences of that change, reflecting on these processes and consequences and then replanning and so on (Kemmis and McTaggart, 2000). In this case Louca-Mai worked with CCHP staff, young people and other stakeholders through a series of workshops, focus groups and meetings in order to explore the systems and processes required for CYP's participation to be embedded effectively.

The project involved two stages: the focus of the **first stage** was the development of a CCHP participation strategy through a series of workshops with staff from the NHS Trust and Barnardo's and young people who had been involved in CCHP participation activity alongside meetings of a core steering group ('core group' in Figure 7.1). Initially the staff and young people's groups met separately in order to consider their different perspectives and experiences of participation and ensure the young people had the support they needed to be confident in contributing in workshops with the adult professionals. We then met together as a whole group to co-design a participation strategy and framework (CCHP, 2016b).

The strategy and framework for embedding participation which emerged from this collaborative process were launched at an event in April 2014, attended by Kath Evans (contributor to this book), then the NHS England Head of Patient Experience for Children and Young People and young people and professionals involved in the project along with commissioners, senior Trust executives, and clinical and Barnardo's staff. The event also included a showing of *Our Participation Story*, a film on the personal benefits of participation made by young

Figure 7.1: CCHP stage 1 process

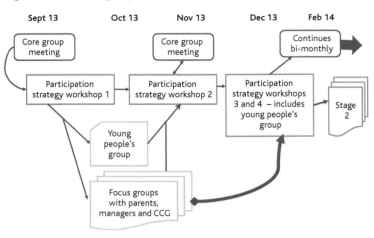

Source: Brady (2017)

people involved in the development of the strategy, facilitated by Barnardo's HYPE service, (CCHP, 2014b).

The core element of the **second stage** was a second action research cycle structured around a series of workshops in which Louca-Mai supported the CCHP Community Paediatric Physiotherapy service to put the strategy and framework developed in stage one into practice, and look at what it meant to 'embed' young people's participation into their service.

At the first workshop with the physiotherapy team we began by considering where people thought they were in embedding participation in their service, where they wanted to be and how they might get there. In between workshops the physiotherapy team tried to put the strategy and framework into practice, working with members of the Barnardo's HYPE team to try and embed participation in their services. In the second and third workshops the group came together to reflect on what had helped and hindered their efforts to embed participation and revise plans. During this second stage, between May and October 2014 there were two meetings of the core group and three workshops with physiotherapy staff, a co-inquiry group with the parents involved in stage one and a focus group with CAMHS professional leads. Alongside the work with the physiotherapy team Barnardo's took forward the young people's request at the end of stage one to develop a poster and film, reporting back at the sharing event discussed earlier. We talked about testing out some of these materials with other young people who may not have had prior experience of participation ('focus groups with other YP' in Figure 7.2) but in the end there was not enough time to do this. Everything was brought together at a meeting in October 2014 (the 'revised strategy' in Figure 7.2). This meeting included updates on work undertaken since the end of the first stage in February 2014 by some of the young people who had been working with Barnardo's and by the physiotherapy team and reflections on emerging learning, the research process and next steps.

Figure 7.2: CCHP stage 2 process

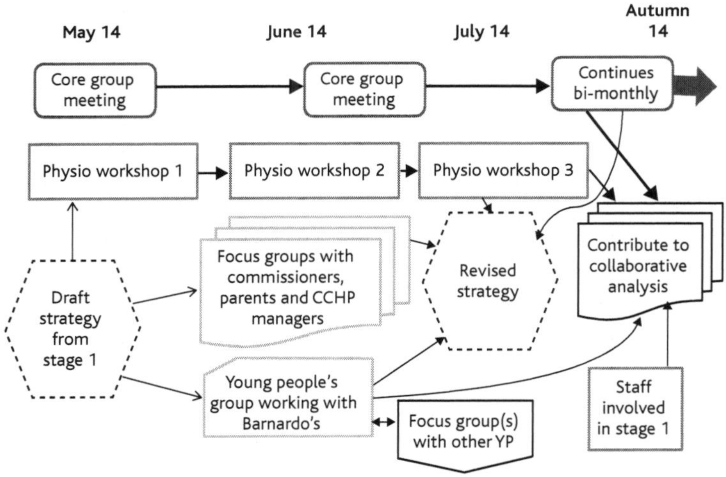

Source: Brady (2017)

Development of the CCHP participation strategy: Louca-Mai's reflections on the process

During my initial discussions with CCHP managers they identified a need to develop a coherent participation strategy in order to create more consistency across services and provide some guiding principles:

'[This] strategy needs to actually set the culture, the ethos, of the organisation.' Health professional

When this approach had been agreed by the staff and young people involved in the stage 1 workshops outlined earlier, we began exploring people's views on what the strategy should look like. Participants agreed that it should set the culture and ethos for participation and focus on values and principles that would be linked to key indicators set out in a related participation framework, along with a leaflet for CYP. The plan was that the draft strategy would be developed during the first cycle of workshops and then finalised by Barnardo's after piloting in the second cycle. Once it was signed off and disseminated, services and areas of CCHP would then be expected to develop a participation plan using the framework and strategy and report back on this. Broadly this is what happened, other than the young people deciding to make a film and poster instead of a leaflet, and the roll-out and dissemination being slowed down by the earlier than expected recommissioning of CCHP (discussed further in the Epilogue).

The final strategy states that the CCHP's ambition was:

> ... to establish participation as an everyday process –
> understood, valued and acted upon by professionals
> and children, young people and their parents/
> carers. The CCHP self-assessment framework of
> participation standards means that services and
> functions can apply this strategy to the work they do.
> CCHP Participation Strategy, p 2 (CCHP, 2016b)

The intention was that the participation strategy and associated framework (Brady, 2017 and Chapter 10) would be a starting point both for the development of participation in CCHP services and, hopefully, a vision and statement of intent for commissioners and potential new contract holders. It was hoped that the associated film (CCHP, 2015b) and other materials developed by young people would similarly raise awareness of participation among current and potential users of CCHP services.

Box 7.2: Lizzy's experience

It was amazing to be a part of creating the strategy right from the start. It challenged me by being in larger groups of people than I was used to. We began meeting as separate groups, one being children and young people (CYP) and the HYPE staff supporting us, and the other group being staff from a variety of CCHP services. We then came together to share views and ideas as a team. It blurred the lines between 'us' and 'them', and I think it helped each of us see that every person involved had something valuable to bring to the discussions. Sharing highlighted that how 'qualified' you were, or weren't, didn't matter within the practice of participation.

At first, I found the whole process quite intimidating, but Louca-Mai and the HYPE staff supporting me ensured that everything was explained in an age appropriate way, and that our voices as CYP were heard. I think for me this felt especially important, because I was so anxious in a group setting that my words wouldn't come easily. I was often too fear filled to speak aloud in front of everyone. Again, Louca-Mai and the HYPE staff made it accessible for me to still participate, by talking with me, and sharing my views for me when I didn't feel able to verbalise them myself.

I found it really interesting to hear so many people's ideas and views on the future of participation in CCHP, and what that might look like. It was exciting discussing how the information could be adapted and delivered to CYP of various ages and abilities, and to staff, to ensure it was easy to understand.

Working on a project about participation, that had participation fully embedded from the beginning was great. It was such a brilliant showcase of how capable and intelligent CYP are, when engaging in serious subjects such as the future of CCHP and matters regarding their healthcare. Being so involved in creating the strategy gave me a bigger insight into the 'behind the scenes' planning that goes into services – which as a YP you'd rarely otherwise get to see.

It was highlighted to me that my experiences in a wide range of CCHP services meant I had a wealth of knowledge and insight that could be a useful resource. I had the ability and voice within me to say about a service "this was great because…" or, on the reverse, "This really didn't work for me, let's improve it." This felt empowering. It's only when you are open to hearing Children and Young People's own experiences and views on their healthcare that you can start to make proactive and positive changes towards the care of future CYP.

At times I found it difficult to concentrate or found information hard to understand and process. It was my job though to voice this, and it was always seen as a positive when I did, because if I was confused, often I wasn't the only one. This meant Louca-Mai could work with us finding different, more user-friendly ways to explain things.

For me, knowing that I could be part of preventing some of the struggles I had within services, for the next CYP coming through them, was the fuel that drove me onwards. Not only did I want to see changes, but I myself could be part of that change.

Box 7.3: Felicity's experience

I used health services for a long period before CCHP was formed and for a short while after. I then remained involved in the capacity of an ex-service user for five years. The width and breadth of my experience has enabled me to witness the changing ethos of participation in health services. Due to the inherent barriers and challenges discussed earlier there was some initial resistance, but over time this was replaced in CCHP by a passion for children's participation at both individual and strategic level[s].

As a group of young people with a collective experience of ten different services within CCHP we knew first hand that pockets of excellent participation were happening in the organisation, but also that the journey was not complete. We wanted to help develop a strategy to embed participation on every level so that all children and young people using CCHP services were having a consistently positive experience. We wanted to give participation the same importance as every other policy and provide a standard and formal tool for professionals to work to.

We met on several occasions with staff from CCHP and this partnership seemed to ignite a lot of enthusiasm and discussion. We tried to work creatively which was somewhat novel for some staff, but really facilitated expression and cohesion and dissolved the disparity between young people and staff. The development of an authentic and meaningful strategy could only have been achieved through authentic and meaningful collaboration – as that was the very essence of what we were aspiring to embed.

When the strategy was written, we worked together with staff to make it come alive, be truly meaningful and become more than words on paper. We also thought about how we communicate to young people what they can expect from good healthcare and what 'good' looks like in relation to both experience of services and participation. Another young person and I worked with Barnardo's to produce a film of our participation journey. The past few years of our lives had been quite a difficult journey. We both agreed that a big part of the progress we have made can be attributed to the participation we have been involved in. We made the film to convey the impact and difference good participation makes to individuals on a more personal level.

Having started out in participation as a service user I am now working as a healthcare professional, and it seems that it is also pretty difficult to enthuse staff about policies from that perspective! If there is a more accessible version hanging around, I find that staff make a beeline for it. I think that the process we went through to create the strategy made it come alive for staff as well as young people. Narratives are a really powerful way to get staff on board, especially when the people who those narratives belong to are sitting right there in the room with you.

Key areas of learning

Understanding participation in practice

We began by exploring how participation was understood by the practitioners and young people involved in the workshops so that we could agree a shared understanding from which to build.

This process highlighted how individual-level participation in health services can help to develop CYP's capacity for more participation in strategy and policy:

> 'People needed to be empowered and feel empowered ... whether that is in their day-to-day care, so they are feeling empowered towards making decisions ... or whether that is acquiring knowledge and experience and skills to take place in other forms of decision-making ... it is about building people's capacity to be included.' Participation worker

Individual participation can also inform the development of services and policy more directly. For example, Barnardo's had worked with parents to gather stories from families of CYP with particular health conditions, which were then used in work on care pathways in order to give clinicians an understanding of people's journey through accessing services, receiving a diagnosis and further involvement from the relevant professional teams, as well as new insights into the 'patient journey' beyond their services.[1]

CYP's participation in the development of policy and services tends to focus on adult-initiated, context-specific participation within a formal setting (Davis and Hill, 2006; Malone and Hartung, 2010) often in formal groups such as forums and advisory groups (Crowley, 2015). But we found that how CYP were involved in the development of policy and practice was as important as what they were involved in. As discussed in Chapter 1 CYP are not a homogenous group and we found that formal participation groups did not work for everyone and assume a model of participation in which CYP have ongoing involvement with an organisation. But many CYP using a health service such as CAMHS, physiotherapy or school nursing would not necessarily identify themselves as a service user of the larger organisation of which the service is a part. We sought to address this through the creation of opportunities for shared learning and tools and practical support to develop both practitioners' and CYP's confidence. Young people involved in the project spoke about the benefits of participation for their wider peer group, as well as personal benefits including being able to use difficult personal experiences to create positive change. However, doing this safely required building relationships of trust with the adults supporting their participation.

We found that good participation, especially in the development of services and policy required expertise and the identification or appointment of specific members of staff 'dedicated to the development of participation' (Wright et al, 2006, p 24). As Barnardo's were not responsible for delivering clinical services they were in a more neutral role and able to be a critical friend, as well as championing participation and taking the lead in developing practice and evaluating participation. But this needed to be balanced with the need to make participation 'everyone's business' and acknowledge CYP as 'experts by experience'. Young people involved in the workshops talked about how participation should be empowering and have benefits for both CYP involved and their wider peers (for example several talked about it helping their recovery), but also about the importance of participation needing to be meaningful and lead to change.

Involving young people in the development of a strategy

The process of involving young people in the development of the CCHP participation strategy and framework highlighted some interesting issues around implementing ideas of participation in the development of policy. The intention was that the strategy and associated framework would be both a starting point for the development of participation in CCHP services and, hopefully, a vision and statement of intent for commissioners and potential new contract holders. An associated film and other materials developed by young people, with support from Barnardo's, would similarly raise awareness of participation among current and potential users of CCHP services. The collaborative nature of the project was seen as really important:

> 'We wouldn't have been able to create [the strategy] without the different types of people who are in this room [and] some people who are not in this

room … there's no way Barnardo's or young people or [CCHP] staff could have done this on their own. It's quite a powerful demonstration to me of how much better things are when you [create] them from different type of perspectives.' Participation worker

But the original plan for a 'one size fits all' strategy for staff and young people changed when it became clear that what was needed for the development of organisational practice would not work for CYP and vice versa:

'[I]t's really difficult to enthuse young people about strategies and policies… It only comes alive when they can relate it to their own experiences and then they … understand what it's about more. Especially from the children's rights angle, a lot of young people get passionate about "oh, we need to make it better for other young people, they don't want to go through the same thing that I went through and we need to change that".' Participation worker

'We [group of young people involved in the workshop] had quite a hard time trying to read through [the draft strategy] … because we felt (it) was too wordy and that the meaning was sort of lost because it was taking so much energy to read all the words … we all thought that maybe the idea of having a poster of the values … re-writing them in a more simple way [would be better], we couldn't … understand how you can only have one version of [the strategy] really, how one version could meet all the needs of staff, parents and young people and we thought a poster would be good and we would have a cool time designing it.' Young person

Having a clear, organisation-wide vision and standards for participation for all staff across the CCHP, and CYP using CCHP services, was central to embedding participation – hence the strategy and framework. But, as discussed earlier in this chapter, CYP using health services may come and go, and talk about seeing a physiotherapist or going to CAMHS rather than identifying themselves as a user of CCHP services. Perhaps this model may work for the CYP who work with the Barnardo's HYPE service in strategic or service-development-related participation activity, but we wanted something that would be relevant to every child coming into CCHP services. Therefore, the materials developed by young people focused on informing CYP about their right to have a say in the services they used, rather than being something to which they needed to 'sign up'. So, what we ended up with was separate but linked documents: the participation strategy and framework alongside the young people's film and poster. Furthermore, this work and events associated with it, created a significant breakthrough in CCHP being able to reach other services and as a result more CYP and families. CCHP also started more diverse informal group opportunities to enable a wider range of CYP to meet and give their participation more flexibility as well as structure.

A culture of participation

A culture of participation is the ethos of an organisation, shared by professionals and young people, in which participation is seen as a wider concept than just specific events or activities (Kirby et al, 2003; Wright et al, 2006). A culture of participation was described by research participants as a process and a journey, as well as a set of shared values that inform practice. In the CCHP, 'culture' and associated attitudes to participation were felt to vary within and between services, professional groups and geographical areas as well as within the wider NHS:

> 'the engagement of [some services in] this process [the collaborative workshops] is a struggle, as the gap in understanding of participation across the partnership is still big ... the majority view [of CYP's participation in the CCHP] tends to be about ... [CYP's] access to services as opposed to your views changing services and your care.' Participation worker

This raised questions about whether and how professionals identified as being part of a larger organisation rather that the specific service in which they worked, and how far a complex and geographically spread out organisation like CCHP could be said to have a 'culture'. We found that it was important to understand professional identities as well as organisational structures and decision-making processes before deciding on the best way to embed participation. Our work with the CCHP was essentially about building on and embedding a participative culture which was a core part of the ethos of the organisation and had relevance to individual services:

> 'How do we ensure that everyone who works in CCHP and uses its services believes that participation is important? ... They'll think it's important if they really understand or believe that it improves the service they can deliver ... [there's] no point just telling people they've got to do it. It just won't work.' Health professional

Leadership and responsibility

A shared commitment to participation needs leadership in order to be developed and supported, including but not limited to management support for participation practitioners, maintaining participation as an organisational priority and addressing resistance to change (Wright et al, 2006):

> '[Participation] has to be engineered to start with ... you are going to need [management] to say "this has to for a period of time be a priority" ... if [participation] isn't one of those things that's being said is important then it will just be drowned out by other targets and commissioners.' Participation worker

While the CCHP had staff at all levels who were very committed to participation and some experienced young champions, it was also a large and complex organisation in which understanding and experience of participation varied considerably. The challenge for embedding was how to maintain it as a priority and provide leadership when faced with restructures and the resulting change and uncertainty.

> 'People go "I haven't got the time, I can't be doing that, someone else will have to do it", but I feel that is the only way that [participation] will really filter in properly is if it really is just embedded in what we do.' Health professional

Participation expertise, skills and champions (both formally nominated and informal) were needed to support the embedding of participation in the CCHP. Champions within services can represent the views of other practitioners, cascading participation and driving implementation as well as potentially being a first point of contact for children and young people. In the case of individual participation this might mean being the person children and young people can go to if they have a concern or complaint about their experience or ideas about how things could be improved. People with in-depth understanding of participation (the 'participation professionals', in this case Barnardo's HYPE staff) helped to ensure that it remained on the agenda in CCHP services, encouraged and supported the sharing of good practice and challenged and developed practice which required improvement:

> '[H]aving Barnardo's ... [as] a voluntary sector pusher, a facilitator, alongside the [Trust] services is absolutely essential. I don't think [clinical services would] have the time and energy to even participate in participation, let alone to drive lead, support, engage with the young people.' Health professional

Participation in healthcare often relies on individual professionals and this can be a barrier to its being embedded in everyday healthcare practice, as well as creating a focus on consultation with children and young people about their individual health needs rather than collaboration in the commissioning, delivery or evaluation of health services (Blades et al, 2013; Ocloo and Matthews, 2016). We found that the role participation professionals needed to play was to facilitate and enable participation rather than being seen as the people who 'do' participation, and there was a need to address tensions between the need for participation champions and expertise and the idea of participation as a collective endeavour in which everyone had a stake.

Epilogue: the impact of recommissioning on embedding participation

Despite the local and national recognition of the participation work supported by Barnardo's in the CCHP, the organisation has since been restructured following a long and complex recommissioning process, which involved a substantial reduction in resources, especially for participation. The CCHP had been in operation since 2009 but, after the initial five-year contract was extended by two years, the way European law is applied in the UK required that the commissioning bodies responsible go through a process of recommissioning. The consultation process for this recommissioning started in 2014 but was delayed and the contract extended again for an additional year, with the new substantive contract planned to be awarded in summer 2016 for an April 2017 start. However, in May 2015 the NHS Trust announced that they had decided not to extend the CCHP contract beyond their contracted date of March 2016, and that they did not intend to bid for the next contract. The main reason given for this was that the Trust felt that their strategic direction required them to focus on acute and hospital-based care and that the CCHP service sat outside this. This announcement caused considerable upheaval and resulted in the commissioning of an interim one year 'lift and shift' contract starting in April 2016 (supporting existing arrangements, performance levels and contracts at the point of transfer). This interim contract was awarded in November 2015 to a partnership of three organisations (two community-based social enterprises and one NHS Mental Health Trust). The CCHP kept its name for the interim year and the lead organisation in the partnership continued subcontracting Barnardo's HYPE service. This meant that the planned roll-out of the participation strategy and framework developed during this study continued to happen, albeit more slowly than had been planned. The re-procurement for the substantive contract started in February 2016 and the Barnardo's element of the service went through a competitive tendering process with project cuts of up to 75 per cent. Bar a workshop to discuss emerging findings in summer 2015 Louca-Mai's active work with the CCHP ended in October 2014, so many of these events happened after the research on which this chapter draws. Nonetheless the recommissioning had an increasing impact towards the end of the project, both for staff and young people. The young people involved in the HYPE service had developed a huge ownership of the participation ethos, and one young person set up an online petition and had a formal meeting with commissioners about their concerns and how unsettling the process was for them. It also had longer-term implications for the embedding of participation in the CCHP.

Following the interim recommissioning in 2016 the CCHP was delivered as an interim partnership between three healthcare organisations and Barnardo's. This new partnership was then commissioned to deliver the new substantive contract, from April 2017 until March 2022, after the full re-procurement process. At the time of writing a separate recommissioning process of Bristol and South Gloucestershire community adult services in 2018 saw two of the social enterprise provider organisations in the partnership become competitors in the bid for these adult services. These two organisations were at that time separately providing these recommissioned adult services. The commissioners decided to merge the contracts for the two local authority areas of Bristol and South Gloucestershire to ensure one provider. The outcome of which was that one of the social enterprise organisations involved in the CCHP partnership was awarded the new adult services contract in 2019 to start in April 2020. The other social enterprise organisation lost their existing adult contract which meant that they were no longer viable, and they therefore gave notice on all their contracts in autumn 2019 including their CCHP services. At the time of writing, the Barnardo's HYPE service had significantly diminished resources, which were stretched very thinly across the myriad of services in CCHP. The impact of this latest wave of change means that service delivery priorities were once more focused on transferring staff, and young people's participation had a more stop start existence within the affected services, challenging the ambition to embed this way of working. In contrast within the CAMHS services where leadership and organisational culture benefitted from continuity, young people's participation had been increasingly embraced with a greater sense that young people's active involvement in their care and service development could be a permanent fixture.

Discussion

Although the CCHP was unique in the way a health and a voluntary sector organisation had come together to deliver a service underpinned by CYP's participation, it has lessons for health services and policy development in the UK and more widely. We found that for participation to be meaningful and effective for both health services and CYP, that participation, and children's rights, need to be embedded in the development and delivery of health policy and practice. This includes a focus on working in child-centred ways and a commitment to developing policy in collaboration with CYP.

Realistic participation in policy and service development requires honest consideration of the boundaries and limits such as wider organisational policies and procedures, requirements of commissioners and regulatory bodies and available resources. CYP's participation and the systems and processes which support this are interdependent, and these internal and external influences can both support and limit CYP's participation in policy and service development. At the same time, it is important to acknowledge and seek to address issues of power and control and consider what say CYP have in what they are participating in, and how, when and where they participate. In order to be effective CYP's participation in health needs to measure both the quality of CYP's engagement in participation and the impact of this process on service quality, improvement and policy. CYP need to see that they are part of an evolving and improving process for them, and services and mechanisms need to be in place to prioritise this alongside other work commitments.

As well as the potential to further develop practice this work also identified the need to capture learning and examples of good and innovative practice which may otherwise be lost. The current climate of austerity and increasing privatisation of NHS services has implications for CYP's participation, particularly when learning from participation is still not routinely captured or shared.

One of the intentions of procurement is to review and improve the health outcomes and experiences for CYP, access to services and the impact the services have on their health outcomes. The recommissioning of CCHP services meant an opportunity was lost to learn more about how the CCHP's innovative approach, and our work on this project, had supported the embedding of participation and the impacts and outcomes of this participation on service design and delivery and children, young people's and families experiences of services.

Acknowledgements

With thanks to all the staff and young people from the CCHP who collaborated on this work, and without whom it would not have happened, and to North Bristol NHS Trust for supporting it. Also, thanks to the University of the West of England for funding the studentship which supported this research, and Barry Percy-Smith and David Evans, Louca-Mai's supervisors at UWE.

Note

[1] http://cchp.nhs.uk/cchp/your-say/cchp-family-stories

References

Beazley, H. and Ennew, J. (2006) Participatory methods and approaches: Tackling the two tyrannies. In V. Desai and R.B. Potter (eds.) (2016) *Doing Development Research*. London: SAGE.

Blades, R., Renton, Z., La Valle, I., Clements, K., Gibb, J. and Lea, J. (2013) *We would like to make a change: Children and young people's participation in strategic health decision-making*. London: Office of the Children's Commissioner. Available from: www.childrenscommissioner.gov.uk/publication/we-would-like-to-make-a-change/

Brady, L.M. (2017) *Rhetoric to reality: An inquiry into embedding young people's participation in health services and research.* PhD thesis, University of the West of England. Available from: http://eprints.uwe.ac.uk/29885

Brady, L.M., Hathway, F. and Roberts, R. (2018) A case study of children's participation in health policy and practice. In P. Beresford and S. Carr (eds.) (2018) *Social Policy First Hand.* Bristol: Policy Press, pp 62–73.

Care Quality Commission (CQC) (2015) North Bristol NHS Trust *Community health services for children, young people and families: Quality Report* [online]. Available from: www.cqc.org. uk/sites/default/files/rvj_coreservice_community_health_ services_for_children_young_people_and_families_north_ bristol_nhs_trust_scheduled_20150211.pdf

CCHP (2014a) *What is the Community Children's Health Partnership?* Available from: http://cchp.nhs.uk/cchp/what-cchp [Last accessed: 11th November 2019].

CCHP (2014b) *CCHP values.* Available from: http:// cchp.nhs.uk/cchp/what-cchp/cchp-values [Last accessed: 11th November 2019].

CCHP (2015a) *Barnardo's HYPE.* Available from: http://cchp. nhs.uk/cchp/what-cchp/barnardos-hype [Last accessed: 11th November 2019].

CCHP (2015b) *What goes on in there?* Available from: http:// cchp.nhs.uk/cchp/visiting-cchp/what-goes-there [Last accessed: 11th November 2019].

CCHP (2016a) *Young people's charter.* Available from: http://cchp. nhs.uk/cchp/your-say/young-peoples-charter [Last accessed: 11th November 2019].

CCHP (2016b) *CCHP children and young people's participation strategy.* Available from: https://cchp.nhs.uk/sites/default/ files/09-HYPE_Participation_Strategy-FINAL-March16-office.pdf [Last accessed: 11th November 2019].

Crowley, A. (2015) Is anyone listening? The impact of children's participation on public policy. *International Journal of Children's Rights*, 23 (3), pp 602–21.

Davis, J.M. and Hill, M. (2006) Introduction. In E.K.M. Tisdall, J.M. Davis, M. Hill and A. Prout (eds.) (2006) *Children, Young People and Social Inclusion: Participation for what?* Bristol: Policy Press, pp 1–22.

Kemmis, S. and McTaggart, R. (2000) Participatory action research. In N.K. Denzin and Y.S. Lincoln (eds.) (2000) *Handbook of Qualitative Research*. 2nd edition. London: SAGE.

Kirby, P., Lanyon, C., Cronin, K. and Sinclair, R. (2003) *Building a culture of participation: Involving children and young people in policy, service planning, delivery and evaluation.* (Report and Handbook) London: DfES.

Malone, K. and Hartung, C. (2010) Challenges of participatory practice with children. In B. Percy-Smith and N. Thomas (eds.) (2010) *A Handbook of Children and Young People's Participation: Perspectives from Theory and Practice.* London: Routledge, pp 24–38.

Ocloo, J. and Matthews, R. (2016) From tokenism to empowerment: Progressing patient and public involvement in healthcare improvement. *BMJ Quality and Safety*, 25 (8), pp 1–7. Available from: http://qualitysafety.bmj.com/content/early/2016/03/18/bmjqs-2015–004839.abstract

Reason, P. and Bradbury, H. (2008) Introduction. In P. Reason and H. Bradbury (eds.) (2008) *The SAGE Handbook of Action Research: Participative Inquiry and Practice.* 2nd edition. London: SAGE, pp 1–10.

Roberts, E. (2016) E-mail to Louca-Mai Brady, 18 February.

Torrance, H. (2011) Qualitative research, science, and government: Evidence, criteria, policy, and politics. In N.K. Denzin and Y.S. Lincoln (eds.) (2011) *The SAGE Handbook of Qualitative Research*. 4th edition. London: SAGE, pp 569–80.

Wright, P., Turner, C., Clay, D. and Mills, H. (2006) Involving *children and young people in developing social care.* Participation Practice Guide 06, London: SCIE. Available from: www.scie.org.uk/publications/guides/guide11/

PART IV

Young people-led participation

8

Investing in Children: respecting rights and promoting agency

*Liam Cairns, Chris Affleck,
Chloe Brown and Helen Mulhearn*

Introduction

Investing in Children (IiC) is an organisation which exists to promote the human rights of children and young people, in particular their right to have a say in decisions that affect them, as defined by Article 12 of the United Nations Convention on the Rights of the Child (UNCRC). We do this primarily by creating spaces in which children and young people can come together, identify and discuss issues, and develop arguments about how these issues might be addressed. IiC then supports them to enter into dialogue with adults who have the power to act on their agenda.

This chapter will draw upon IiC's archive of work over the last 22 years, along with testimony from young people involved in two of our current projects: Type 1 Kidz, an initiative for young people with Type 1 diabetes, and YASC, a youth café providing support to young people transitioning from CAMHS (Child and Adolescent Mental Health Services) to Adult Mental Health Services, to inform a discussion on the nature of *effective* engagement in dialogue, and the relevance and significance of IiC's collaborative approach. In particular, we will consider the notion that participation is not a single event (or a series of events) but a sustainable process through which children and young people are seeking to take effective action on issues which they identify as in need of change. It is this clarity about the purpose of participation which lies at the heart of the IiC approach.

In Section 2 we consider some of the complexities of creating opportunities for children and young people to be seen as genuine contributors to dialogue about decisions that affect them, and how focus on the *process* of participation without critical attention on the *purpose and intended outcomes* of participative practice has resulted in confusion.

In Section 3 we describe the origins of IiC, and how the IiC practice model developed, highlighting a key point at which the contribution of children and young people changed the direction of the organisation by helping us to appreciate the difference between consultation and active participation.

In Section 4 we consider three case examples, one from our archive and two from our current range of projects, where the participants have gone on to become active agents in creating new solutions to the dilemmas that they faced.

Finally, in Section 5, we consider whether it is the quality of IiC's relationship with the children and young people with whom we work, and our willingness to be led by them that, on occasions, has created the circumstances where it has been possible to move beyond participation in dialogue to agency.

Creating meaningful participation

Muscroft described the broad vision of the UN Convention thus:

> Children are seen as full human beings, right-holders who can play an active part in the enjoyment of their rights. They are not — as they have often been presented in the past — mere dependants, the property of their parents. They are not people who only become full human beings when they become adults. They are in need of protection but also have strengths. Every child is seen as important, no matter

what its abilities, origins or gender. Their views and opinions are significant. They are not to be seen merely as victims, workers, young offenders, pupils or consumers, but as complex and fully rounded individuals. (Muscroft, 1999, p 16)

Designing a process through which the genuine and meaningful participation of children and young people is secured requires careful thought. The UN Committee on the Rights of the Child defines participation as 'ongoing processes, which include information sharing and dialogue between children and adults based on mutual respect, and in which children can learn how their views and those of adults are taken into account and shape the outcome of such processes' (UN Committee on the Rights of the Child, 2009). This is a relatively passive definition, in which the primary objective would appear to be the creation of learning opportunities for children and young people.

In an article discussing the various benefits of young people's participation, Sinclair notes the need for 'greater honesty about the purpose of participation activity and whose agenda it is serving' (Sinclair, 2004). In 2003, IiC contributed to an ESRC research project that considered the link between children's participation rights and social inclusion. This proposed a more active and ambitious definition of the purpose of participation:

- Participation is about ensuring that the voices of children and young people are heard. Practice needs to be focused upon creating opportunities for engagement in dialogue between children and young people and decision-makers.
- Participative practice should be concerned with the lived lives of children and young people. Practice needs to be concerned with issues that young people agree are important to them.
- Participation needs to be understood as a means to a political end. As with any other group in society, children and young people will participate in political debate in order to make things better. Participation is part of a process of seeking to take effective action.

- Participative practice needs to be inclusive. The key is to create opportunities for children and young people to participate on their own terms, and not simply to satisfy the expectations of the adult community.
- Participation needs to be transformative. In other words. It needs to challenge the dominant discourse that represents children and young people as lacking the knowledge or competence to be participants in the policy debate. (Davis and Edwards, 2004)

This definition, and in particular the observation that participation is 'part of a process of seeking to take effective action', is the definition that IiC has embraced. IiC sets out to create opportunities that are based upon *participative* (or *assertive*) rather than *representative* models of democratic engagement (Williamson, 2014). The children and young people who contribute to IiC projects do so on their own behalf, and not as representatives of others. This approach has created space for the views of many children and young people who are rarely included to be heard and taken into account. It has allowed these children and young people to say what they want to say and 'participate on their own terms, and not simply to satisfy the expectations of the adult community'. As a consequence, as Williamson has remarked:

> A consultative, representative model of how to involve young people in decision-making does not lead to situations where mainstream institutions or their managers feel challenged to change what they do and how they work. Investing in Children almost invariably will challenge them for it brings into the open perspectives that might otherwise remain in the shadows expressed as grumbling and dissatisfaction rather than as something to be openly debated and changed. (Williamson, 2003)

Although children and young people's right to be seen as legitimate participants in decisions that affect them is guaranteed in Article 12 of the UN Convention on the Rights of the

Child, the extent to which this has been embraced in practice is debatable (Lundy, 2007; Stalford and Drywood, 2009; James, 2011). While there is some evidence of a change in rhetoric, it is less easy to provide evidence of a change in the extent to which the participation rights of children and young people are respected in reality. Arguably, some of the mechanisms that have been adopted are ineffective, that is, they create an impression of participation without the contribution of children and young people having any actual impact upon the outcome of the debate (Shenton, 1999; Crimmens, 2005; Henricson and Bainham, 2005; Mori, 2005; Cairns, 2006).

This is the political reality in which we live. The dominant discourse on childhood condemns them to a peculiarly vulnerable position within society. The representation of children and young people as objects of adult concern, or works in progress, or naturally unruly and in need of control and socialisation, but seldom as competent agents and citizens with rights effectively confines them to a state of political impotency (Cairns, 2006). The inherent weakness in IiC's attempts to ensure that 'participation is part of a process of seeking to take effective action' is that the power to act often lies with adults who are not inclined to listen. Although there are now a number of significant examples where we have supported young people to achieve genuine change, it remains the case that these are the exception rather than the rule.

In the face of adult indifference, most often young people shrug and move on – you could argue that their expectations are realistically low. But on occasions, young people have taken the initiative and created change for themselves, and in Section 4 we consider three case studies that highlight this. However, it must be acknowledged that creating genuine opportunities for children and young to be seen, as Muscroft proposes, 'as full human beings, right-holders who can play an active part in the enjoyment of their rights' (1999, p 16) by having their voices heard in a way that results in change is by no means easy, and the power differential between adults and children is so great that it is unsurprising that we fail more often than we succeed in supporting children and young people to achieve the change that they seek.

The origins of Investing in Children

IiC was created in the mid-90s in County Durham, in the North East of England, by managers in the local authority and the National Health Service (NHS), in an effort to improve the accessibility of services used by children and families, by ensuring that agencies adopted a more integrated approach to service delivery. It was proposed that the UN Convention on the Rights of the Child (CRC) provided a framework of values and principles which could be agreed as underpinning both joint and separate operations. The working group charged with the responsibility of designing a process to achieve this ambition proposed the adoption of the following:

Box 8.1: Investing in Children Statement of Intent

Our aim is to work in partnership with children and young people to promote their best interests and enhance their quality of life.

We will achieve this by:

- consulting with children, young people and their families about decisions affecting their lives and the development of services;
- promoting partnerships between individuals and agencies to address young people's issues;
- developing accessible children and young people and family-centred services that promote dignity and independence and which do not discriminate or stigmatise;
- ensuring that, when making decisions on policies and services, consideration is given to their potential impact on the lives of children and young people.

The values that underpin our work with children and young people are consistent with the UN Convention on the Rights of the Child and the Children Act 1989.

Durham County Council, 1995

IiC became an operational project in 1997. The purpose of the project was to 'explore and address some of the issues thrown up by the adoption of these principles and values. It was acknowledged that the realisation of the vision of the Convention as previously described would require a radical change in the way we think about children, and in the way children and young people are treated, particularly by the key institutions concerned with them' (Cairns et al, 2005).

One of the first projects undertaken by IiC was the drafting of the Children Services Plan for County Durham. This was a policy document which outlined the integrated arrangements made by the local authority and its partners, to provide services for children and their families. Given the IiC Statement of Intent which made explicit our commitment to children's rights, considerable effort was made to consult with a wide range of children and young people, and a substantial section of the final document was given over to their views.

At a public event to launch the Plan, partner agencies expressed their satisfaction with the work we had done and, in particular, with the way that we had included the voices of children and young people. However, one of the young people who had been consulted effectively rained on our parade by commenting: "I'm not interested in your grand plans and strategies. I want to know – can you help me change things where I live my life?" (Cairns, 2001).

This was a turning point for IiC and had a profound effect on the organisation's future. It led us to understand that participation needs to be seen as a means to an end, as part of a political process of seeking to take effective action, and not an end in itself.

IiC works to create spaces in which children and young people can come together, discuss issues and develop ideas about how things might change. This is achieved through supporting young people to run 'Agenda Days' and assisting them to research items on their agenda, in preparation for entering into dialogue with adults who may have the power to act upon their proposals. An Agenda Day is a tool developed by IiC to enable large (15–30) groups of children and young people to explore issues and create an agenda for action (hence the name). Essentially an Agenda Day provides an adult-free environment in which participants can share experiences, exchange ideas and come up with possible actions. Agenda Days are facilitated by young people who have previous experience of the approach, who will record the debate and create a draft report. This is then circulated to all participants for their endorsement. Within some common-sense considerations (for example, Agenda Days for very young children require consent and often collaboration from parents and carers) Agenda Days are open events.

Agenda Days often lead to the formation of Research Groups, where young people spend time researching issues and refining their arguments, before attempting to enter into dialogue with adults who may have the power to make change. Evidence from IiC's work over the last 21 years clearly demonstrates that, given the opportunity, children and young people are knowledgeable about the world in which they live, and can be powerful participants in political dialogue and persuasive advocates on their own behalf (Williamson, 2003; Davis, 2007).

As noted earlier, the weakness in this approach is that the power to act on the arguments presented by young people often rests with adults, some of whom have been unwilling to enter into the dialogue. However, when dialogue is achieved, even where it is tentative to start, the results can be impressive as the following case studies illustrate.

Case studies

Club Idol

In the early days of Investing in Children, we worked with a group of young people who were dissatisfied with the social and leisure facilities available to them in the ex-mining town in East Durham where they lived. To add insult to injury, they were also frustrated by the fact that they were often 'moved on' by the police when they met their friends in the street, even though, as they observed, there was nowhere else to go.

Investing in Children supported the young people to conduct research by running Agenda Days and eventually, to take their findings to the local Community Safety Partnership, who were in the process of producing a Youth Strategy.

The main findings of the young people's research were:

- There was very little leisure provision for young people in the area. Many of the facilities that young people might choose to use (pool hall, bowling alley, cinema and so on) were not available in the district, and travelling outside the district to access them is difficult because of high transport costs. Local facilities (McDonald's, the leisure centre and so on) were seen to be inhospitable (that is, they did not make young people welcome). Inevitably, many young people spend time socialising in groups, on the street.
- This causes its own problems: "Well over half the young people said they feel safe at the places they socialise. This is due to the fact that they are in large groups and feel safer than they would if they were on their own. However, the police don't like young people being in groups, so they move us on or split us up." (Plant et al, 2002)
- Stereotyping of young people. There was a *strong* feeling that attitudes towards young people were strongly influenced by negative stereotypes. For example, young people hang about outside a local convenience shop which stays open late into the evening. They are aware that their presence there is seen as a problem: "This can cause problems, as some old people feel intimidated by large groups of young people. Old people ... seem to think every teenager is a thug." (Plant et al, 2002)
- Respect. "We are always hearing about how young people have no respect for adults or for property and so on. Well, how about a bit of respect for us?" From the police to leisure centre staff to employees of McDonald's and Boots the Chemist, young people provided examples of how they were treated with suspicion and a lack of respect. (Plant et al, 2002)

When the Community Safety Partnership published their Youth Strategy, the young people were disappointed (although not surprised) to learn that their contribution had been all but ignored. They decided that they would continue to argue their case. They were aware that the local leisure centre was so poorly frequented on Friday evenings that it often closed early. So they approached the manager of the centre, and proposed that they would run a regular music event for young people in the centre on Friday evenings, to be called 'Youth Idol'.

What followed was a difficult negotiation with the leisure centre manager, the local youth service and the police, that went on for a number of months. Without dismissing the proposal out of hand, the adults wanted to set boundaries that the young people believed to be so onerous that they would sink the project before it had even started. For example, the leisure centre manager wanted to limit admission to those who had paid a hefty membership fee. The local police inspector wanted to know what plans the young people had to ensure that there would be no substance abuse at the event and that participants would be kept safe, and the youth service were insistent that youth workers should be involved the running of the club.

The young people held their ground. They argued that the price of admission was a key issue, which, if set too high, would effectively exclude many of their friends, and insisted that the charge should be modest enough to be within the limited budget of their peer group. They said that the presence of the police would be a major deterrent for many young people who had an uneasy relationship with officers. They persuaded the police inspector that the private security guard who patrolled the outside of the building, and who, they pointed out, was in radio contact with the nearby police station was adequate security, and that they (the young people) would accept responsibility for internal arrangements. They pointed out that many young people chose not to attend the existing local youth clubs provided by the youth service, largely because the service's commitment to delivering a curriculum of health and safety advice (substance abuse guidance, sex education and so on) made the clubs too much like their experience of school. The compromise reluctantly proposed by the young people was that a youth worker could attend on condition that the worker refrained from interfering or offering unsolicited advice.

Eventually, their arguments were accepted. Club Idol was a huge success, regularly attended by over 100 young people, with no notable incidents. One of the young people involved offered his explanation of the project's success:

> 'When we did Club Idol it worked because young people were involved every step of the way and when the adults raised the problem of a charge to get in, the solution was suggested by the young people. They wanted it run by adults, but the young people weren't for that and they organised it themselves, designed the posters, proper security like a club at every stage – it worked and they had a hundred young people coming regularly.' (Davis, 2007)

However, reflecting one of the other inherent challenges to sustaining an active and vibrant children's rights strategy, when the original creators outgrew the club and moved on to other things, attendance gradually dropped, and the club closed (Cairns and Brannen, 2005).

YASC

In recent years, support for children and young people's mental health and emotional wellbeing has been coming under increased pressure, with a rising number of referrals to organisations like the CAMHS. As a consequence, there can be a significant wait for an assessment. In County Durham and Darlington around 30 per cent of referrals to CAMHS are signposted to other services, but only after an assessment has been completed. Early intervention and preventative services are severely limited, which means that many young people aren't getting the support they need to develop the resilience and acquire the coping mechanisms that will help them with the situations they find most challenging (Moore and Gammie, 2018; YoungMinds, 2018).

In 2015, IiC were asked to create spaces for children and young people to come together and contribute to a review of CAMHS Service being conducted by the two Durham-based

Clinical Commissioning Groups (CCGs). At the same time, IiC was assisting children and young people and their families to contribute to the development of the Children and Young People's Mental Health, Emotional Wellbeing Resilience and Local Transformation Plan (LTP).

To facilitate this process, a series of Agenda Days was arranged, involving a range of children and young people including: young people who identify as LGBTQ (lesbian, gay, bisexual, transgender, queer); looked after children and young people (children and young people in the care of the local authority); young people accessing mental health support services; and young people with special educational needs and disabilities.

Two reoccurring themes were identified by children and young people who attended these events:

- the lack of opportunities for informal peer support for young people struggling with their mental health and emotional wellbeing;
- and the difficulty some young people experience during the transition from Children's to Adult services.

After a series of meetings with the young people who had facilitated the Agenda Days which identified this serious gap in service availability within County Durham, Waddington Street Resource Centre, an Adult Mental Health facility, agreed to work with the young people and IiC to explore ways to plug this gap. Young people recommended that an art project would provide a positive focus and a means of expressing feelings and emotions without having to talk about them. IiC and the Resource Centre committed to deliver a ten-week pilot project.

One of the main unforeseen successes of the project was the development of social groups formed by previously socially isolated young people, who began to meet up prior to the art group to go out for a coffee. In discussion with the young people, IiC and the Resource Centre began to explore ways of extending the offer to young people who had no interest in art. This then led to another pilot project in the form of an informal drop-in café which opened prior to the art group.

This project, now known as the Young Adult Support Café (YASC) has proven to be a real success. In addition to providing a safe space for young people to access informal peer support, YASC enables young people to smoothly transition from Children and Young People's services into Adult services. In addition, YASC works in partnership with a range of organisations and services to signpost young people to opportunities that enable them to progress into education, employment, training and volunteer work.

This is one of the key achievements (and was one of the main objectives) of the group – to support the smooth transition from Children's to Adult services. By the end of 2017, six of the regular attendees of the group who had reached the upper age limit had been successfully supported either into an adult service or into an alternative group. One of the benefits of the YASC being located within the Resource Centre is that a number of the young adults are now able to access daytime services provided by the centre, which has provided additional support to their transition into Adult services.

In 2018, YASC supported young people to link in with supported internships through the NHS and helped a number of young adults to access daytime services and courses through Adult Mental Health Services. In addition, a number of young people have signed up to do voluntary work with children and young people through IiC, or with adult clients of Waddington Street Mental Health Centre. Due to the quality of her work on a Comic Relief funded Investing in Children Social Action programme, another young person joined the IiC pool of paid sessional workers.

In September, five members of the group moved on to university. For two of these young people, university was always part of their plan, although mental ill-health issues had created some uncertainty. It is a significant achievement for this group to have moved from being socially isolated to accessing regular mental health services to taking up university courses. One of the group is studying to become a mental health nurse.

One of the participants in the project agreed to record her experience. This is what she had to say:

Box 8.2: Rowan's story

I found out about the group through a friend. At the time I was struggling with social anxiety and low mood, so I was barely leaving the house. My friend suggested I go with her to help me get out more. The group has a wonderful range of activities, usually from 5pm to 6pm, it's mostly chatting and catching up with people, something I used to find quite daunting, though it's fine if you're not up to talking much. Then there's the option to go to the art room which is lovely as if you're not sure what to do, people can suggest things to make or draw. I love seeing everyone's artwork and it has really helped me get over my fear of drawing in front of people. There is also a quiet room if you need a quiet place to be/calm down. Sometimes there are themed nights, I really enjoyed Halloween as there was an opportunity to dress up. There are also board, card games and film nights.

Going to this group has helped me so much, from social interactions to getting back into a routine. I've met so many lovely people and made some really good friends after not being able to cope meeting new people.

What's good is knowing you won't be judged, the sheer amount of support from everyone, knowing that I'm less isolated and that there are others who are also going through things – oh and the frequent offers of a hot drink!

I would recommend YASC because it has completely changed my life around and been a large part of getting better, and I haven't heard of anywhere else like this. I think it fills an important space for young people who need support, might be struggling, who are interested in art or just need somewhere to go.

I just want to say thank you and hope the group can continue helping more people.

Type 1 Kidz

This project has its origins in the early days of IiC.

Around 300 children and young people under the age of 18 are currently living with Type 1 diabetes in County Durham and Darlington. Type 1 diabetes is a life-long autoimmune condition which cannot be prevented and has no cure.

In 2001, children were typically diagnosed with the condition between the ages of 6 and 10. They immediately had to start testing their blood and taking multi-daily injections which has a significant impact on quality of life on the young person and the family as a whole. As Type 1 diabetes is so complex it requires careful management from a Paediatric Multi-Disciplinary Team, which in 2001 included consultants, specialist nurses, dieticians and healthcare assistants. Patients were expected to attend an appointment at least every three months. However, many families weren't engaging well with the specialist team, and as a consequence young people were not controlling their diabetes well at home. Statistics showed that the North East of England was falling behind the rest of country, increasing the risk of both short- and long-term complications for the health of children and young people.

The Lead Consultant from the Paediatric Multi-Disciplinary Team approached IiC and asked if we could start a project to find out why children and young people weren't engaging and how the service could change the way they operate to better support families. This was the beginning of the project that would eventually become Type 1 Kidz (Cairns and Brannen, 2005).

A small group of children and young people with diabetes were recruited who facilitated a number of Agenda Days in which a much larger group contributed their experiences of the health services used by them and made suggestions about how these could be improved. As a result, a number of changes were made: a psychologist was employed as part of the clinical team; the structure and timing of clinics were altered; and children and young people assumed responsibility for updating notice boards with appropriate material.

Throughout these discussions, children and young people and their families talked about the need for a peer support project that would provide a place where people with similar experiences could come together. As diabetes affects the whole family, they said that a holistic approach was needed. Eventually, this was created, and named Type 1 Kidz.

The project was so successful in County Durham and Darlington that other Health Trusts approached IiC, and in 2014, Type 1 Kidz was extended to a further four areas of the North East – Gateshead, Newcastle, Sunderland and South Tyneside.

The children and young people were clear about what they wanted to achieve by being involved in the project: to feel more empowered to have a say; to be more confident in managing their diabetes; to feel more positive about the future; and ultimately to improve their health outcomes.

Young people lead the sessions. Members of the clinical teams attend the groups and are 'invited' to join discussions by children and young people. A strong relationship between families and clinical teams has developed, resulting in more focused and specialised care, and an open forum where new ideas and suggestions are shared and discussed. The IiC Project Worker also has a close relationship with all of the clinical teams and attends the County Durham and Darlington Multi-Disciplinary Team meeting to ensure that communication flows between the clinicians and the families, and that nothing is missed.

As a result, family engagement has been high. Two hundred and eighteen families have engaged in sessions, an average of 20 per cent of the patient population; in one Trust 46 per cent of their patients have attended a session. Families report that they feel more confident and positive about the future and can evidence changes that have happened as a result of being involved in the project. Local teams have also changed their ways of working with children and young people and some have completely altered their approach to the conduct of appointments. For example, after a discussion with 10–11-year-olds in Newcastle, the team now encourage children and young people to lead their appointment by reviewing their own diabetes management and suggesting what changes should be made to their medication, rather than the team telling them what to do (Brown and Mulhearn, 2017, Mulhearn and Brown, 2017).

Here are the views of two young people and two parents who have been involved:

Box 8.3: Holly's story

I was diagnosed with Type 1 diabetes when I was nine years old, on 30th December 2017. I was shocked as there were no history of the disease in my family. I was introduced to Type 1 Kidz the day I was discharged from hospital. The first time I went to Type 1 Kidz I felt like I wasn't different to anyone else, unlike I did at school and any other public place, even at home. Along with this, I found out about insulin pumps and CGM's and now I have an Omnipod and Dexcom G6 of my own this improves my quality of life because I don't need to think about it as much. I am now included in fun activities and days out including residential trips I now also have more self-confidence than I did before I started going to the group. Because of this, my diabetes doesn't really affect me any more, or at least not as much as it did. If I described it to another child they would probably think it is just a common club like what they go to but trust me, it's life-changing and it really is. I feel like it could change other lives as well and not just mine. I am now not ashamed of my condition not even nearly as much as when I was diagnosed that I truly feel like everyone should experience that amazing, once in a lifetime feeling.

Box 8.4: Ben's story

I was diagnosed with Type 1 diabetes when I was only 11 months old. I am now 14, so I have had diabetes for as long as I can remember. I was the only one in my primary school with Type 1, so I had never met another person with my condition until I was about eight, when I started coming to t1kz. This is a group of children and young people who meet together monthly and we do things such as sports and games for example dodgeball. We also do some work to improve life in the local area, for children and young people with Type 1, such as improving waiting rooms and hospital services. From coming to t1kz I have learnt a lot about how others manage their diabetes. For example, you can see others using technology such as the Dexcom which monitors our glucose and warns the user and parent if your blood sugar is too high or too low, because of t1kz I have now started using this and it has given me much better control of my diabetes.

I was asked to talk at the Centre for Life to children who have been recently diagnosed and their parents. We discussed leaflets and different services and with the parents we also discussed their hopes and fears for the future. The feedback from this was very positive.

We also recently went on a residential visit to Duke's House Wood, where we did many fun activities such as high ropes and the 3G swing. It is a great opportunity to meet new people who go through the same things that you do and share your own experiences of the Type 1 diabetes that you both have to live with and manage every day. We have also done a lot of work with Newcastle airport to improve services there for people with Type 1, as we have to wear equipment that could fail to work if it goes through the airport security scanner, however, airport staff are not trained on this, so sometimes pressure people with Type 1 to go through the body scanner, which Is very dangerous. This happened to me last year and might discourage families with newly diagnosed children to go on holiday for the first time. I have also had the opportunity to speak in a boardroom meeting to GPs about what it is like living with Type 1, in order to give them a better insight into the condition, which will help their patients, as Type 1 is often misdiagnosed like I was.

Box 8.5: A parent's comment

Type 1 Kidz is an absolute life and sanity saver. The group has given so much support to both adults and the children. As a parent of two Type 1 kids we have all benefited so much from these groups.

Box 8.6: A parent's comment

Type 1 Kidz isn't just a group for kids, it's an invaluable support for carers too. Soon after diagnosis, when it can feel that you are drowning in information, seeing other children just being 'normal' and listening to other parents explaining that 'the whirlwind of emotions is to be expected', can be incredibly reassuring. Along with advice from our clinic, it helped us understand our options and helped us come to the right decision about the path we wanted to go down. Now, over six months in, it still feels just as important to connect with other T1 families. The benefits of having that opportunity to connect with other T1 families can't be over-stated and, as a parent, I have to say I feel we benefit from it just as much as my son.

Discussion and conclusions

We would suggest that these three very different case studies, to a greater or lesser extent, have a number of things in common:

- In all three cases, the children and young people were *agents* in creating responses to the challenges they faced. They took the initiative and did not wait for the adults to solve their problems.
- The projects took time to develop, and the children and young people showed patience and resilience, drawing strength from a growing sense of solidarity.
- The projects that were created were based upon their ideas. In the case of Type 1 Kidz and YASC, the role of the adults was to provide support and assistance as they turned their ideas into action. This was also eventually the case with Club Idol, although the process was more conflictual.
- The children and young people retained a leadership role when the projects became operational.
- Their motivation appears to be a mixture of self-help and the desire to make life better for others who face the same challenges.

A certain amount of confidence was required to achieve the progress that was made. Self-confidence, certainly in the case of Club Idol, but also confidence in IiC, and a belief that we would support them to make their case and work with them to find solutions. This begs the question: how does IiC command such confidence?

We believe that part of the answer lies in the way that we attempt to build relationships with the children and young people with whom we work. The following are the key elements of our approach:

A *rights-based approach*

Children and young people have rights, including the right to have a say in decisions that affect them. Many of the young people with whom we work have little or no previous knowledge or experience of this, and exploring this provides the starting point for most of our projects. We explain that the principal purpose of IiC is the promotion of their right to be heard. This is a matter of social justice, and we are committed to supporting them to exercise their right, and if necessary, to challenge situations in which adults unreasonably refuse to listen to what they have to say.

We have some evidence of the impact that this has. In 2014, in an ESRC-funded project called 'Looking Back', a researcher interviewed young adults who had been involved with IiC in their teens. In her report she noted that:

- Several participants said that they had little knowledge of their rights before being involved with Investing in Children.
- While many participants did not directly use the term 'rights', they spoke of being increasingly aware of injustices in the world and the importance of making their voices heard.

The participants in the study told her:

> *"(Investing in Children) makes you aware as a young person you actually have a right to a voice."*

> *"Makes you feel like your voice is heard because it's you saying what you want to happen."*

> *"I think that when you look at other organisations and how they work with young people and then look at Investing in Children it's clear they're just that bit different to how*

everybody else is because they do listen, they do try to act upon what the young people are saying rather than just ticking the boxes saying 'we've listened to them.'"

"They're going to listen to you and whatever they say they'll do their best to try and put into action, they like listen to young people and resolve problems." (Maynard, 2014)

Honesty

Bill Williamson has considerable knowledge of IiC, having conducted an early evaluation of the project. He commented:

> Initiatives in this domain often do not achieve the changes that young people may have identified at the outset. Although Investing in Children has achieved some notable successes, there are many more examples where projects have not resulted in effective dialogue. This is part of the political process. Experience suggests that children and young people are as capable of understanding and dealing with political reality as any other group. We must strive to continue to support young people to seek new, more effective strategies, but the fear of failure must not be used as an excuse for inaction. (Williamson and Cairns, 2006)

We believe that it is important that we are honest and open about this, and at the beginning of every new project we make it very clear to children and young people that we cannot guarantee that the change they are seeking will be achieved.

Respect

IiC strives to 'walk the walk as well as talk the talk' by treating the children and young people with whom we work with respect which we believe they deserve from others. The 'Decisions Group' consisting of young people from all of the existing projects, scrutinises the work of the IiC team. In addition, when we left the County Council in 2013 and became a cooperative Community Interest Company, we created a Board of Directors that provides equal representation to the three parties who form the enterprise. Three seats are allocated to our commissioners, three to members of staff and three to young people.

Two further comments from external studies of IiC:

'The IiC workers are amazing, they are not discriminating at all, they treat people with equal rights and really listen to you and they are more kind of sit back, let you have your and kind of not push in. And it learns you how to stand up for yourself and for the future.' (Davis, 2011, p 93)

In a similar vein, one of the contributors to the Looking Back research commented:

'The staff were always on a ground level, you never felt as though they were better than you. They are very approachable and treat young people as individuals and respect their opinions and most importantly listen and give children and young people a voice. I felt very empowered while working with Investing in Children.' (Maynard, 2014)

Conclusions

We believe that IiC has developed a distinct approach to promoting the rights of children and young people, one in which children and young people themselves play a significant role. We define the task of the organisation in explicitly political terms, measuring our effectiveness in terms of the extent to which genuine change is achieved.

We have had some notable successes, some of which have involved supporting children and young people to go from being advocates arguing for change to become agents in the creation of new ways of working, as the case studies presented demonstrate.

But the political reality is that the power differential between adults and children is so wide, and the dominant discourse that defines children and young people as lacking in the knowledge, experience and ability to participate in political debate is so strong that we fail more often than we succeed. Yet children and young people continue to enthusiastically attend Agenda Days and enlist in campaigns. We believe that our sustained relevance is derived from the quality of the relationships that are fashioned through our approach, which is based upon the clarity of our aims, our frankness about the scale of the challenge and the environment of mutual respect that we strive to maintain.

If there are lessons here about the future development of children and young people's participation in the design and delivery of health services (or indeed any other public service), we would suggest that paying attention to clarity about the purpose of participation is much more important than process or structure. We would suggest that the proposed definition produced by the ESRC research project, outlined in Section 2, is a good place to start. If a service's participation strategy is focused on addressing the challenges contained in this definition, it is likely to resonate with a wide range of children and young people and create the circumstances where their engagement will be both easy to secure and sustained.

References

Brown, C. and Mulhearn, H. (2017) The Type 1 Kidz project. Part Two: Introducing a simple telehealth system. *Journal of Diabetes Nursing*, 21, 32–5.

Cairns, L. (2001) Investing in children: Learning how to promote the rights of all children. *Children & Society*, 5 (5), pp 347–60.

Cairns, L. (2006) Participation with purpose – The right to be heard. In E.K.M Tisdall, J.M. Davis, M. Hill and A. Prout (eds.) *Children, Young People and Social Inclusion: Participation for What?* Bristol: Policy Press, pp 217–34.

Cairns, L. and Brannen, M. (2005) Promoting the human rights of children and young people. The 'investing in children' experience. *Adoption & Fostering*, 29 (1), pp 78–87.

Cairns, L., Williamson, B. and Kemp, P. (2005) Young People and Civil Society: Lessons from a Case Study of Active Learning for Active Citizenship in D. Wildemeersch, V. Stoobants and M. Bron Jr (eds) *Active Citizenship and Multiple Identities in Europe*. Bern: Peter Lang.

Crimmens, D. (2005) The role of government in promoting youth participation in England. In D. Crimmens and A. West (eds.) *Having their Say: Young People and Participation: European Experiences*. Lyme Regis: Russell House.

Davis, J. (2007) *University of Edinburgh evaluation of investing in children. Final report.* Internal Investing in Children Archive. Unpublished.

Davis, J. (2011) *Integrated Children's Services*. London: Sage.

Davis, J. and Edwards, R. (2004) Setting the agenda: Social inclusion, children and young people. *Children & Society*, 18, pp 97–105.

Durham County Council (1995) *Investing in children. A consultation paper*. Durham: Durham County Council.

Henricson, C. and Bainham, A. (2005) *The Child and Family Policy Divide*. York: Joseph Rowntree Foundation.

James, A. (2011) To be (come) or not to be (come): Understanding children's citizenship. *The ANNALS of the American Academy of Political and Social Science*, 633 (1), pp 167–79.

Lundy, L. (2007) 'Voice' is not enough: Conceptualising Article 12 of the United Nations Convention on the Rights of the Child. *British Educational Research Journal*, 33 (6), pp 927–42.

Maynard, N. (2014) *Looking Back. Investing in Children Project Pack*. University of Durham.

Moore, A. and Gammie, J. (2018) Revealed: Hundreds of children wait more than a year for specialist help. *Health Service Journal*, 30th August 2018.

Mori, L. (2005) Young people as outsiders: The Italian process of youth inclusion. In D. Crimmens and A. West (eds.) *Having their Say. Young People and Participation: European Experiences*. Lyme Regis: Russell House

Mulhearn, H. and Brown, C. (2017) The Type 1 Kidz project. Part 1: Engaging children and young people with type 1 diabetes in their own health and wellbeing. *Journal of Diabetes Nursing*, 21 (1), pp 28–31.

Muscroft, S. (ed.) (1999) *Children's Rights: Reality or Rhetoric?* London: International Save the Children Alliance.

Plant, O. et al (2002) *Growing up in Peterlee*. Internal Investing in Children Archive. Unpublished.

Shenton, F. (1999) *Evaluation of County Durham's 'Investing in Children' initiative*. Durham: University of Durham.

Sinclair, R. (2004) Participation in practice: Making it meaningful, effective and sustainable. *Children & Society*, 18 (2), pp 106–18.

Stalford, H. and Drywood, E. (2009) *Coming of Age? Children's Rights in the European Union*. European Children's Rights Unit. Liverpool: University of Liverpool.

UN Committee on the Rights of the Child (2009) The Right of the Child to be Heard, General Comment No 12 (http://www2.ohchr.org/english/bodies/crc/docs/AdvanceVersions/CRC-C-GC-12.doc)

Williamson, B. (2003) *The grit in the oyster. Evaluation of Investing in Children*. Durham: University of Durham.

Williamson, B. and Cairns, L. (2006) *Working in partnership with children and young people Report of a Research in Practice Conference*. Internal Investing in Children Archive. Unpublished.

Williamson, B. (2014) *Discussion Paper. A Democratic Approach to Education*. Internal Investing in Children Archive. Unpublished.

YoungMinds (2018) Available from: https://youngminds.org.uk/blog/new-figures-on-camhs-waiting-times/

9

RAiISE: advocating for young people with invisible illnesses

*Sophie Ainsworth, Jenny (Sammy) Ainsworth,
Robyn Challinor, Jennifer Preston, Marie Clapham,
Laura Whitty and Simon Stones*

Introduction

In this chapter, we discuss RAiISE (Raising Awareness of invisible Illnesses in Schools and Education), a charity founded in the United Kingdom that is led by young people, for young people. From the perspective of the Chief Executive Officer (CEO) and the Board of Trustees, all of whom have lived experience of invisible illnesses themselves or as a parent/carer, we will provide insight into day-to-day life for the charity and its unique journey from an initial idea of one young person diagnosed with a chronic health condition to a national organisation with a global presence. RAiISE is a positive example of young people leading health and wellbeing initiatives with the support of healthcare and education professionals, rather than *simple* instances of young people's engagement or involvement. It also highlights the importance of collaboration across sectors, including schools and charities, to ensure that young people with health conditions are adequately supported, acknowledging the wider impact of health on a young person's life – away from the hospital. In this chapter, we will refer to 'invisible illnesses', which for context, is an umbrella term for any health condition that isn't easily visible to others. This includes chronic conditions such as cystic fibrosis, diabetes, inflammatory bowel diseases and musculoskeletal diseases, among others – but also mental health illnesses such as anxiety, depression and schizophrenia. RAiISE attempts to be as inclusive as possible in reference to invisible illnesses and equally helps to place the spotlight on visible illnesses affecting young people too.

What matters to us: young people's perspective on participation in healthcare

The importance of young people's involvement in healthcare is undeniable, and recent years have shown a positive increase in the inclusion of young people's voices in decision-making processes in healthcare (Weil et al, 2015). While there are discussions in both child and adult healthcare, it is important to acknowledge that there is no distinct line or 'cut-off' between childhood and adulthood, and the ways in which these groups engage with healthcare, despite organisational and legal definitions of who is defined as a child or adult. Therefore, the 'young person' demographic must have a place to voice their own unique experiences and concerns of healthcare, which indeed differs from younger children and older adults with health conditions (Betz et al, 2013). Across healthcare and research, there is a tier of different roles in which young people interact with services and health research (Table 9.1). Examples of such activities include membership of youth forums such as RCPCH &Us from the Royal College of Paediatrics and Child Health (RCPCH, see Chapter 4), GenerationR Young People's Advisory Groups, social media takeover days and involvement in hospital trusts and clinical commissioning groups. Meanwhile, the discussion of how to involve young people in research, and to what extent, continues to be a source of debate among the research and clinical community (Davies et al, 2019), often due to a lack of awareness and capacity to undertake robust and thorough involvement (Preston et al, 2019). A framework was published in 2019 to aid the design and review research

Table 9.1: Examples of young people's participation, engagement and involvement in healthcare services and research

	Participation	Engagement	Involvement
In the context of healthcare services	When young people take part in shared decision making about their health in partnership with their healthcare professionals. *For example, young people discuss with their doctor which treatment is least likely to cause side effects.*	When information about healthcare services are shared with young people. *For example, informing young people about how to book appointments with their GP* online.*	When young people are actively involved in shaping healthcare delivery and services. *For example, in co-designing a new adolescent clinic.*
In the context of research	When young people take part in a research study. *For example, completing a questionnaire study.*	When research knowledge is shared with young people. *For example, outreach via social media and science festivals.*	When young people are actively involved in shaping a research study as a research partner. *For example, setting research priorities for young people with a certain invisible illness.*

*GP = General Practitioner.

involving young people by setting out a series of Questions and Considerations to answer (Phillips et al, 2019).

RAiISE is unique in that it was founded by a young person and continues to be run by a management team of whom half are young people. This structure is essential in embedding the issues which can only be accurately identified by those with lived experience of being a young person with health conditions in the 21st century. RAiISE supports young people with health conditions in a variety of ways, but its core focus is on schools. Principally, how health conditions can impact a young person's education and what schools can, and should, be doing to help. RAiISE advocates for a holistic approach to the management of health conditions, uniting the young person, their families, healthcare professionals and schools together to secure the best outcomes for young people. This approach enables us to highlight the problems which health conditions may cause for young people and where more support may be needed. We feel it is important to highlight the impact of health conditions beyond the clinic; after all, young people generally spend a comparatively small amount of their time within the hospital environment. When assessing disease activity, young people may well feel it is more appropriate to record patient-reported outcomes over clinical outcomes when attempting to understand how a young person is doing. In other words, biomarkers and laboratory tests don't necessarily paint the full picture of how well a young person is doing; though understanding that their condition is preventing them from going out with their friends can show the real situation an individual is in. Similarly, the school can greatly impact both physical and psychosocial outcomes for young people, depending on the kind of support available to them. School-related stress has a large impact on many young people, which can be hugely increased for young people with health conditions. Academic support, exam concessions and general empathy, understanding and leniency from school staff can alleviate stress for young people with health conditions in education. Only by engaging with young people with chronic conditions about their daily life outside of the clinic can healthcare professionals identify and help to resolve such issues.

Addressing the need for better support for young people with invisible illnesses in education

Chronic health conditions as a whole are the leading causes of death and disability worldwide, with estimates suggesting that between 13 and 27 per cent of young people live with one or more conditions (Wijlaars et al, 2016), many of which are often 'invisible'. In the UK, this equates to one in seven young people aged 11–15 (Hagell et al, 2013). These conditions affect various aspects of young people's lives, from challenging misconceptions to fighting inequalities within education as previously alluded to, despite legislation enacted to ensure that young people (and adults) with health conditions are not discriminated against. However, this is not what is often observed in practice and the consequences can endure into adulthood. Therefore,

RAiISE feels that action is needed to empower and educate young people with health conditions to realise their potential while supporting them to feel confident in their ability to self-advocate. In addition, professionals involved in the care and education of young people need to be motivated to be inclusive in the present and mindful of their role in preparing young people for their future.

Establishing RAiISE – Raising Awareness of invisible Illnesses in Schools and Education

The need for RAiISE emerged directly from the experiences of Sophie Ainsworth, who would go on to establish RAiISE. After her diagnosis with Juvenile Systemic Lupus Erythematosus (JSLE) at the age of 14, Sophie endured a great number of difficulties at school. These were largely due to a lack of awareness about the nature of health conditions like JSLE, and the profound impact these conditions have on young people. In the months after her diagnosis, Sophie began to conceptualise what would eventually evolve into RAiISE, motivated by her negative experiences. During one of her appointments at Alder Hey Children's Hospital NHS Foundation Trust, Sophie shared her ideas with Consultant Rheumatologist Eve Smith, who connected Sophie with the Patient and Public Involvement Manager within the Alder Hey Clinical Research Facility, Jenny Preston. These early, informal conversations led by Sophie, with the support of professionals, initiated the foundations of RAiISE.

Identifying unmet needs and priorities

Between October 2015 and March 2017, three expert stakeholder workshops were hosted in Liverpool to develop the initial concepts of RAiISE, which at that point was known as the 'Invisible Illness Project'. By networking with contacts she had developed, Sophie identified 30 young people who were interested in the project. During the first workshop held in October 2015 (Preston and Ainsworth, 2015), four young people and two parents were in attendance. During the two-hour workshop, co-facilitated by Sophie and Jenny, young people shared what it was like to live with a health condition, including feelings of isolation, low self-esteem, frustration, unhappiness and guilt when they were accused and ridiculed for being lazy – by both their peers and staff, who failed to understand their individual needs (Figure 9.1).

When asked about support needs, young people highlighted several strategies that could be useful for them individually, and other young people with health conditions more generally. These included: i) a mentor who young people could trust; ii) practical help such as access to lifts; iii) an open dialogue between young people and teachers; iv) education about health conditions within the personal, social, health and economic education (PSHE) curriculum; and v) encouraging teachers to have faith and trust in young people with health conditions.

Participants in the first workshop highlighted several priorities to take forward, which included: i) hosting a workshop with young people, teachers and parents/carers to discuss the issues from the first workshop further; ii) developing an online forum for young people with health conditions to chat with each other about their experiences and concerns; iii) developing information about what it is like living with health conditions; iv) developing a resource for teachers to support young people with health conditions; and v) empowering young people to

Figure 9.1: Expressions of what it is like to live with a health condition as a young person

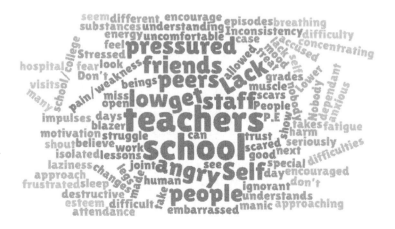

deliver training to schools about supporting young people with health conditions (Figure 9.2). Interestingly, this workshop was the first time many young people with health conditions had voiced their feelings, and they felt that raising awareness of these issues would undoubtedly ease the burden for other young people (Preston et al, 2016).

Following on from the first workshop, an online survey was disseminated via social media to identify the needs and priorities of a wider group of young people with chronic health conditions. Seventeen young people with various conditions completed the survey. When asked how their illness affected them, the most common symptom experienced was fatigue. When asked how their illness affected their life at school, attendance was the top issue, followed by impeding their ability to complete work to deadlines, reducing their concentration, impacting on their ability to cope with exams, restricting their mobility and impacting on friendships. When asked whether they felt that people treated them differently, 41 per cent felt they did. Young people acknowledged that this was most likely due to a misunderstanding of their illness:

- *"you don't look ill"*;
- *"treated as the ill kid"*;

Figure 9.2: Identified strategies to inform and empower teachers and other young people

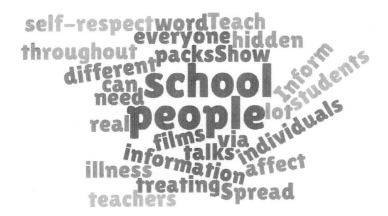

- *"assume I can't do things"*;
- *"both overestimating and underestimating me"*.

When asked whether young people felt staff in school were supportive of them, 71 per cent of respondents said they did, providing examples of how they had been supported in school. These included: exam support; reassurance from school that health should always be their priority; having permission to leave lessons without questioning; support with catching up on work; and having teachers who were empathetic and approachable. Of those who hadn't experienced such positive support in school, examples of what didn't help included: a focus purely on assessment outcomes; poor communication between staff; overlooking information from the young people, their families and healthcare professionals; and forcing young people to do things that were beyond their capacity as a result of their condition. Suggested strategies identified by young people to improve support in school included: learning support; exam support; extensions on work deadlines if required; the ability to leave lessons early without questioning; fast track in queues; and access to lifts when they were unable to take the stairs. When young people were asked if they thought there was enough information about their illness aimed at other young people and school staff, 94 per cent felt there wasn't (Preston and Ainsworth, 2016).

Refining priorities and establishing a resource specification

These responses informed the agenda of a second, larger workshop with a wider group of stakeholders in April 2016 (Preston and Ainsworth, 2016). These stakeholders included young people with health conditions, parents/carers, teachers and healthcare professionals. The aim of this workshop was to begin the phased development of an education resource to improve the way in which young people with health conditions are supported in school. The phased development included: i) assimilating the unmet needs previously identified; ii) developing a resource specification; and iii) designing and refining the resource components and contents.

Participants in the workshop were split into different groups to undertake a series of different activities, which included: i) drafting Top Tips; ii) identifying existing support; iii) suggesting communication methods; and iv) designing a logo and choosing a name for the project. Groups were initially split by stakeholders: young people, parents/carers and teachers. Young people felt that a number of 'Top Tips' needed to be highlighted around effective communication, practical issues and respect (Figure 9.3).

Figure 9.3: Contributions towards the 'Top Tips' for young people, addressing effective communication (a), practical issues (b) and respect (c)

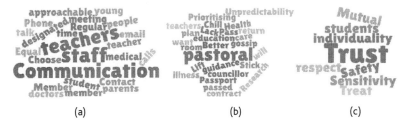

(a) (b) (c)

Teaching staff also highlighted the need to work closely with school nurses and improve consistency in regular staff briefings about young people with health conditions. The importance of the Special Educational Needs Coordinator (SENCO) acting as a liaison between school, home and the hospital was highlighted as an important factor in facilitating support, but it was felt this is inconsistent, particularly within secondary schools. From the parent/carer perspective, key issues and concerns revolved around attendance, exclusion from participating in activities and a lack of consistent and coordinated communication (Figure 9.4).

Parents/carers then discussed some of the solutions for these issues, building on those previously identified from the first workshop. These included:

- *communication between staff* facilitated by a dedicated individual, such as the SENCO, a member of the pastoral staff, or the school nurse, who can bridge communication with home, hospital and school, while cascading information internally;

Figure 9.4: Key concerns and issues expressed by parents/carers

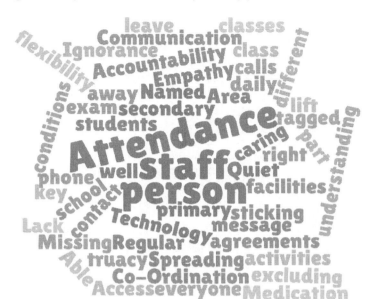

- *practical support* including summaries held by young people which are updated regularly, exit strategies from classrooms, and access to lifts;
- *coping with illness flares and keeping on track with progress*, through the provision of work sent home and deadline extensions;
- *approaching and interacting with young people*, by informing school staff about communicating and dealing with young people who have health conditions, and the impact that may have on behaviour, concentration and socialising. This should include discussions away from other young people, with an attitude that will encourage young people to disclose how they are feeling more openly;
- *empowering young people to inform school staff about their condition.*

After discussion, it was agreed that the components of the education resource would broadly include generic guidance applicable to multiple health conditions, health passports, access passes, health and wellbeing plans, and building accessibility products, among other items.

Identifying appropriate communication methods

In terms of communication methods, a variety of different concepts were discussed. For young people, age and developmentally appropriate games and information were suggested, while assemblies, workshops and teacher training conferences were suggested as ways in which teachers and other school staff could be informed. Information delivery was suggested to be delivered both physically in the form of packs, as well as virtually through websites, social media and e-mail. An important consideration was to ensure that communications remain 'real', with cases and examples from young people, their families and teachers embedded throughout.

Developing the project name and logo

As part of the second workshop, young people were tasked with identifying a name and logo for the project. Several names were suggested, but the final consensus was RAiISE, short for **R**aising **A**wareness of **i**nvisible **I**llnesses in **S**chools and **E**ducation. Draft sketches of logos are shown in Figure 9.5a, with the final sketch shown in Figure 9.5b. During the third workshop in March

Figure 9.5: Draft sketches of the RAiISE logo, designed for and by young people

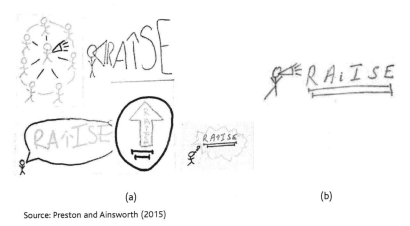

(a)   (b)

Source: Preston and Ainsworth (2015)

2017, the components and content of the education resource were further refined, alongside branding.

It soon became clear that RAiISE was much more than a project, though the resource pack evidently became an integral and important first project for RAiISE. Through networking at various conferences and events (Table 9.2), Sophie identified a team of people to help deliver RAiISE's vision (Figure 9.6). Over a period of two years, the RAiISE management team continued to develop the education resource, while preparing for registration with the Charity Commission. RAiISE was officially registered on 15th November 2018 as a Charitable Incorporated Organisation in England, Number 1180704. As part of the charity registration process, the RAiISE management team developed a constitution, along with a number of supporting strategies and governance documents. These included RAiISE's three core strategic objectives:

- to inform and support schools to help young people with invisible illnesses;
- to empower young people to take control of their health and wellbeing;
- to raise awareness of invisible illnesses in young people.

Figure 9.6: The RAiISE management team

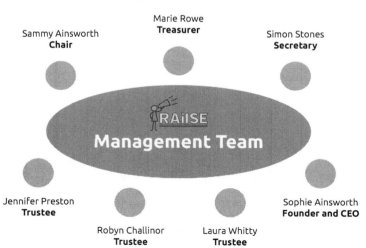

Wider activities and involvement

As RAiISE continues to invest time and effort into internal projects, RAiISE has also reached out to a wide number of organisations to establish positive working relationships under a shared vision of improving the health and wellbeing of young people with health conditions. RAiISE has been visible at a wide range of conferences and events (Table 9.2), including a stakeholder scoping workshop for the National Institute for Health and Care Excellence (NICE), at the outset of developing guidelines for social and emotional wellbeing in primary and secondary education (Stones et al, 2019). RAiISE has also been recognised for its work through various regional and national awards.

Table 9.2: Exemplar conference and events which RAiISE have been invited to attend

- Annual UK Clinical Research Facilities Network Conference (Ainsworth et al, 2018).
- Department for Education meeting.
- European League Against Rheumatism (EULAR) Annual European Congress of Rheumatology.
- European Network for Children with Arthritis (ENCA) Conference
- International Children's Advisory Network (iCAN) Research and Advocacy Summit (Preston et al, 2017).
- National Institute for Health and Care Excellence (NICE) Stakeholder workshop for the social and emotional wellbeing in primary and secondary education guidelines (Stones et al, 2019).
- Paediatric Rheumatology European Society (PReS) Congress (Ainsworth et al, 2017).
- Royal College of Paediatrics and Child Health (RCPCH) Conference and Exhibition (Preston et al, 2016).
- RCPCH State of Child Health report launch in the Palace of Westminster.

Reflections on young person-led initiatives

RAiISE has provided opportunities for young people, their families, and professionals across healthcare, research and education to be active contributors in transforming educational support for young people with health conditions. The phased and pragmatic approach has demonstrated the ability of young people to lead on co-designing products with all relevant stakeholders. This embodies the key principles of co-production, through reciprocity, the sharing of power, including all perspectives, respecting and valuing everyone's knowledge, and by building and maintaining relationships (Hickey et al, 2018). Indeed, RAiISE exemplifies how user-led research and activities can be achieved when young people are supported to navigate through complex environments. The key to this has been in the shifting of responsibilities and the transfer of ownership into the hands of young people, with them forming partnerships with other stakeholders with relevant experience.

Regarding RAiISE's education resource project, the resource pack will be used as part of a pilot study undertaken in a sample of schools in the North of England to assess the feasibility and acceptability of the resource. This project has enabled young people, their families, and professionals involved in the care and education of young people with health conditions to be actively involved in constructing the foundations for rigorously developed resources to inform future practice within schools for young people.

A constant challenge for RAiISE is challenging the public perception of invisible health conditions in young people, by resolving unnecessary misunderstanding and discrimination. We recognise this won't change overnight and will require a long-term and sustained commitment to educating, informing and empowering people to be more open and empathetic towards others. RAiISE actively undertakes activities at the grassroots level; however, influencing policymakers, regulators and inspectors will be a key challenge, especially in overhauling the school assessment system. Moving forward, the health and wellbeing of young people with health conditions must be incorporated into school inspection criteria, such as the 'personal development', 'behaviour and attitudes', and 'schools' leadership and management' judgements (Ofsted, 2019). Given that criteria judgements are being updated, RAiISE feels it's an ideal time to influence such change. It is not our aim to criticise education providers; rather support and inspire positive change for young people – everyone has the right to a happy and good-quality education. RAiISE's movement to better supporting young people with health conditions is not just a current investment in young people, but a longer-term investment in the education, health and wellbeing of our future adult citizens.

RAiISE has always, and will always be, led for and by young people, with the support and encouragement of families, health professionals, researchers, teachers and charities. This is one of the only ways that we are truly going to see a change that benefits young people. Their voice matters, and it is their voice that the rest of us must support. RAiISE is an organisation that is passionate, driven and has big ideas. We want radical change, and we want it now. We want the focus to be on collaboration and breaking down barriers, which can be achieved when we stop doing things the way that they've always been done and start stepping out into the unknown.

Find out more about RAiISE

For more information about RAiISE, please visit: www.raiise. co.uk and contact RAiISE on: info@raiise.co.uk. Don't forget to follow RAiISE on social media as well: @raiiseuk.

Acknowledgements:

Special thanks go to everyone who has been involved in RAiISE since it was founded. In particular, Eve Smith (Alder Hey Children's Hospital NHS Foundation Trust) for her support and encouragement to pursue this initiative, as well as other staff at Alder Hey Children's Hospital NHS Foundation Trust. All of this would also not be possible without the young people, parents/carers, teachers, healthcare professionals and other volunteers who have attended workshops, supported fundraisers and have provided a helping hand to RAiISE.

References

Ainsworth, S., Ainsworth, J., Preston, J., Stones, S.R., Challinor, R. and Rowe, M. (2017) Introducing RAiISE – Raising awareness of invisible illnesses in schools and education. *Pediatric Rheumatology*, 15 (s2), p 113.

Ainsworth, J.S., Ainsworth, S., Challinor, R., Rowe, M., Preston, J. and Stones, S.R. (2018) Things get solved when you become involved: A case study of RAiISE, a young person and family-led research initiative to improve education support for young people with chronic conditions. Poster presentation at: *14th Annual UK Clinical Research Facilities Network Conference*, 12–13 July 2018, Leeds, UK.

Betz, C.L., Lobo, M.L., Nehring, W.M. and Bui, K. (2013) Voices not heard: A systematic review of adolescents' and emerging adults' perspectives of health care transition. *Nursing Outlook*, 61 (5), pp 311–36.

Davies, H.T., Phillips, B., Preston, J. and Stones, S. (2019). Making research central to good paediatric practice. *Archives of Disease in Childhood*, 104, pp 385–8.

Hagell, A., Coleman, J. and Brooks, F. (2013) *Key data on adolescence 2013*. London: AYPH.

Hickey, G., Brearley, S., Coldham, T., Denegri, S., Green, G., Staniszewska, S., Tembo, D., Torok, K. and Turner, K. (2018) *Guidance on co-producing a research project*. Southampton: INVOLVE.

Ofsted (2019) *The education inspection framework*. Manchester: Ofsted.

Phillips, B., Davies, H.T., Preston, J. and Stones, S.R. (2019) Framework to help design and review research involving children. *Archives of Disease in Childhood*, 104, 601–4.

Preston, J. and Ainsworth, S. (2015) *Invisible Illness Project – Part 2 workshop summary report*. Alder Hey Clinical Research Facility.

Preston, J. and Ainsworth, S. (2016) *Invisible illness young person's focus group summary report*. Alder Hey Clinical Research Facility.

Preston, J., Ainsworth, S., Smith, E. and Wilson, E. (2016) G137 Living with an invisible illness. *Archives of Disease in Childhood*, 101 (s1), A73.

Preston, J., Ainsworth, S., Challinor, R. and Stones, S.R. (2017) RAiISE: Raising awareness of invisible illnesses in schools and education. Poster presentation at: *3rd iCAN Research and Advocacy Summit*, 10th–14th July 2017, Orlando, FL, US.

Preston, J., Stones, S.R., Davies, H. and Phillips, B. (2019) How to involve children and young people in what is, after all, their research. *Archives of Disease in Childhood*, 104, pp 494–500.

Stones, S.R., Ainsworth, S., Ainsworth, J.S., Preston, J., Challinor, R. and Rowe, M. (2019) Identifying items for consideration under the remit of the National Institute for Health and Care Excellence (NICE) guideline on social and emotional wellbeing in primary and secondary education. Online poster presentation at *NICE Guideline Stakeholder Workshop for Social and Emotional Wellbeing in Primary and Secondary Education*, 26th March 2019, London, UK.

Weil, L.G., Lemer, C., Webb, E. and Hargeaves, D.S. (2015) The voices of children and young people in health: Where are we now? *Archives of Disease in Childhood*, 100 (10), pp 915–17.

Wijlaars, L.P.M.M., Gilbert, R. and Hardelid, P. (2016) Chronic conditions in children and young people: Learning from administrative data. *Archives of Disease in Childhood*, 101, pp 881–5.

10

Rhetoric to reality: the need for a new approach

Louca-Mai Brady

Drawing together the range and diversity of material included in this book is a challenge which highlights a key message: that one size or form of participation does not fit all. Traditional structures and processes of participation can, at times, be helpful but can potentially exclude some of the young people most likely to use health services and limit the potential for fundamental change. The range of different models and approaches to young people's participation in healthcare practice presented in this book highlight both how 'traditional' structures and approaches can be developed in ways that consider inclusion and diversity, and the potential for new approaches which do more to transfer power to young people.

This chapter concludes the book by drawing together the following themes and issues which emerged from the examples of practice discussed in Chapters 1 to 9, and the research which underpins this book (Brady, 2017):

- defining participation
- cultures of participation
- the changing landscape
- the need for flexibility
- a children's rights-based framework for embedding participation in practice

Defining 'participation'

There is a lack of information on how participation is understood by those who work with children and young people in healthcare, or how these understandings may affect participation cultures and practice (Brady, 2017). The starting point for this book was the commonly held understanding of participation as 'a process by which young people influence decisions which bring about change in themselves, their peers, the services they use and their communities' (Participation Works, 2010, p 9). But while this definition implies a more active form of participation than just listening to children and young people's views, it does not imply a fundamental change in the relationships between young people and service providers (Davis, 2011). In NHS services, as elsewhere, it tends to be adults who do the asking, the listening and have the power to put into practice (or not) decisions which young people are involved in making (Brady et al, 2018). As Cairns et al argue in Chapter 8:

> the reality is that the power differential between adults and children is so wide, and the dominant discourse that defines children and young people as lacking in the knowledge, experience and ability to participate in political debate is so strong that we fail more often than we succeed.

Cairns et al go on to argue that 'paying attention to clarity about the purpose of participation is much more important than process or structure'. The contributors to this book demonstrate that understandings of participation cannot be taken for granted but need to be developed and reviewed, in collaboration with young people, in light of experience and the context in which participation is taking place (Brady, 2017). Understandings of participation inform culture and practice, and exploring these understandings can help to move away from participation being seen only as young people 'having their voices heard' or 'sharing their views', towards more democratic process involving collaboration, dialogue and co-inquiry/co-production to challenge and change systems and practices (Percy-Smith, 2016).

Individual, strategic and collective participation

Participation incorporates two key dimensions: individual and strategic, concerned with *what* young people are involved in; and individual and collective: concerned with *how* young people are involved. We revisit these dimensions in the framework in Figure 10.1, however, it is important to note these are not distinct dimensions, and indeed this book illustrates it is helpful if the boundaries between them are flexible to enable young people to move between levels and types of participation at different points, as well as to develop participation practice which works effectively within organisational cultures, systems and processes. For some young people individual participation is a way to build their capacity to be involved in more strategic or collective participation; for others participation at a strategic level enables them to gain confidence to have a say on an individual level. But, that said, these distinctions between individual, strategic and collective participation are adult constructs which, while important in participation theory and practice, are not necessarily meaningful or important distinctions for the young people involved (Brady, 2017).

Cultures of participation

An important thread that runs through this book is the importance of having culture of participation: an ethos, shared by professionals and young people, in which participation is seen as a wider concept than just specific events or activities (Kirby et al, 2003; Wright et al, 2006). As well as understanding how participation is conceptualised, we need to understand how organisational and socio-cultural contexts inform participation in practice (Tisdall et al, 2014). For example, in Chapter 1 Martin and Feltham discuss how shared decision-making in child and adolescent mental health services is significantly constrained by the ways in which systems and processes privilege the management of risk over the views and choices of young people. In Chapter 6 Percy-Smith et al highlight the need for 'structures, systems and practices for integrating children and young people's views and experiences into strategic decisions making and using learning from that to inform change'. A culture of participation can be seen as a process and a journey, as well as a set of shared values that inform practice (Brady, 2017). But in practice defining a 'culture' of participation is not straightforward in NHS organisations – the lack of consistent approaches or shared values within and between services, professional groups and geographical areas as well as within the wider NHS is highlighted by many contributors to this book. Many NHS organisations are complex and geographically spread out and, as discussed later in this chapter, the voluntary sector and other external agencies also often play a key role in supporting participation. It is therefore important to understand professional identities as well as organisational structures and decision-making processes, and the needs and wishes of young service users, before deciding on the best way to embed participation within a health service or organisation, as well as addressing the cultural tensions discussed in the Introduction between medical models of treatment and understandings of participation and children's rights.

Expertise and champions

A shared commitment to participation needs leadership in order to be developed and supported, including but not limited to management support for participation practitioners and leads, maintaining participation as an organisational priority and addressing resistance to change (Wright et al, 2006). As Whiting et al point out in Chapter 3 effective participation requires financial backing and senior level support as well as expertise 'on the ground'. This is echoed by Percy-Smith et al (Chapter 6), who attribute success in engaging young people in a hospital Trust to 'the hard work and dedication of a small number of staff for whom children's participation falls within their brief'. Participation expertise, skills and champions (both formally nominated and informal) are key to the effective embedding of participation in practice. Champions within services can represent the views of other practitioners, cascading participation and driving implementation as well as potentially being a first point of contact for children and young people. People with in-depth understanding of participation (the 'participation professionals') help to ensure that it remains on the agenda, encourage and support the sharing of good practice and challenge and develop practice which requires improvement (Brady, 2017). For example, in Chapter 3 Whiting et al highlight the importance of the development of trust between healthcare professionals and young people, as well as the role of youth organisations in championing participation and developing good practice. But, as discussed in Chapter 7, it is also important for participation professionals and leads to be seen as the people who facilitate and enable participation rather than the only people who 'do' it. There is a need to address tensions between the need for participation champions and expertise and the idea of participation as a collective endeavour which is everyone's responsibility. Young people can and should be participation champions too, as discussed in many chapters of this book, not least Chapters 8 and 9 on young people-led participation. But it is important to consider the power and influence young champions really have in practice, so that it does not become an exercise in 'window dressing'. This involves consideration of the motivations of and benefits for young champions and exploring with them how they can most effectively be involved in creating change (Brady, 2017).

The role of parents, carers and support services

Young people's participation often includes adults, either parents and carers or professionals, who may as act as 'gatekeepers' and have the power to both enable and constrain young people's participation (Hood et al, 1996; Cree et al, 2002). Healthcare professionals and parents play a significant role in whether and how young people's efforts to participate are facilitated and supported in healthcare settings, and many have reservations or concerns about young people's active participation (Coyne, 2008; Brady, 2017). The dominant model in health services is still one in which the 'consultation takes place between a health professional and the parent as a proxy for the child' (Redsell and Hastings, 2010, p xiii). It is important not to conflate young people's and parents' participation but to see parents and carers as a related but separate group to young people; their views should also be heard as service users but alongside rather than as a proxy for young people's participation. It is also important not to conflate parent and carers' participation as service users or members of the public in their own right with their role as gatekeepers to and enablers of young people's participation. This is powerfully illustrated by Picton-Howell in Chapter 2 in relation to the participation of both parents and disabled young people in end-of-life decisions.

The role of the voluntary sector has been central to the successful participation of young people in many examples discussed in this book including the work of Common Room's Open Talk programme in promoting shared decision-making in mental health services (Chapter 1); the role of the British Youth Council in the NHS Youth Forum (Chapter 3); a partnership between an NHS Trust and Barnardo's children's charity (Chapter 7); the work of the Association for Young People's Health (Chapter 5) and Investing in Children (Chapter 8) in promoting diverse and inclusive approaches to young people's participation in healthcare; and the young people-led work of RAiISE (Chapter 9). Furthermore, there can be advantages to participation being embedded in an organisation, service or project as a parallel process rather than being wholly integrated (Brady, 2017). In Chapter 7 Brady et al discuss the advantages of a voluntary sector organisation sharing responsibility for participation with an NHS Trust: providing participation expertise but with the autonomy to be 'critical friends' without responsibility for the delivery of clinical services.

The changing landscape

The Introduction to this book outlined how paediatric services are seen as the 'poor relation' to adult services within the NHS (Evans, 2016), with the result that NHS care typically results in worse patient experience and lower-quality care for children and young people than for adults (Hargreaves et al, 2019; Viner et al, 2017). The NHS Long Term Plan:

> specifically refers to 'intensifying the NHS's focus on children's health' (3.2) and sets out 'new action to improve the health and wellbeing of children and

young people' (3.7) … [it] includes a commitment to create a Children and Young People's Transformation Programme to oversee the delivery of the commitments to children and young people (3.42). This includes an aim '… to move towards service delivery models for young people that offer person centred and age appropriate care for mental and physical health needs, rather than an arbitrary transition to adult services based on age not need' (3.47). (AYPH, 2019, p 1)

But, while this is encouraging, Chapter 7 illustrates the challenges that procurement and recommissioning processes, along with the increasing break-up and privatisation of NHS services, present to embedding a culture of participation in NHS services. A key challenge for embedding participation in such circumstances is how to maintain it as a priority and provide leadership when faced with change and uncertainty. The NHS Long Term Plan (NHS England, 2019) sets out major changes to the delivery and commissioning of NHS services. Sustainability and Transformation Partnerships (STPs) have been created to bring local health and care leaders together to plan around the long-term needs of local communities. It is expected that by April 2021 every STP will become an Integrated Care System (ICS), through which NHS organisations will plan and deliver services. ICSs will be groups of local NHS organisations working together with each other, local councils and other partners. The NHS Long Term Plan states that every ICS will have a partnership board with commissioners, NHS and voluntary and community sector representatives and 'other partners'. But there is no explicit mention of whether these 'other partners' will include members of the public, let alone specific groups such as children and young people, or of any mandatory requirements for participation, public involvement or engagement in local commissioning beyond talk of ICSs and Clinical Commissioning Groups (CCGs) needing to work with and consult patient groups and voluntary sector organisations working with patient populations. The NHS England Patient and Public Participation Policy (NHS England, 2017) states that 'those responsible for commissioning should be aware of the organisation's statutory duty to involve the public in this area of work and take action as appropriate' (p 15). But STPs were devised largely without public involvement, giving rise to widespread concerns about service loss and concerns about a lack of local accountability or an obvious place for citizen engagement in the 'new NHS' (Hudson, 2018).

Most participation of young people related to the NHS Long Term Plan thus far has focused on participation at a national level, for example through the NHS England Youth Forum (see Chapter 3), the Royal College of Paediatrics and Child Health (RCPCH, 2019) and the Association for Young People's Health (AYPH, 2019). Given the concerns outlined earlier regarding adult involvement this is something that is likely to affect children and young people's participation even more. As Kath Evans says in the Foreword to this book '... policy drivers ... [such as] the NHS Constitution, The Health and Social Care Act, the NHS Long Term Plan, all act as our compasses. Our challenge is to bring these to life'. An important area for future study will be how the changing NHS landscape affects cultures of participation and the young people involved: who is involved, how and the impacts and outcomes of that participation.

Documenting participation

As discussed in the Introduction, while there is growing awareness of the case for children and young people's participation across the NHS in the UK and more widely, there is limited evidence on how this apparent commitment to participation and children's rights translates into professional practice and young people's experience of participation in health services. Given the ongoing changes in the NHS, including post-COVID-19 (see postscript in the Introduction), and the impact of recommissioning of services discussed earlier, it is important to document both what is planned and what happens in practice. A lack of critical reflection, robust evaluation and sharing of learning means that when organisations change, projects end and people leave, knowledge and expertise can be lost.

Critical appraisal of participation is about looking critically at the purpose, consent, method and interpretation of participation in practice (Todd, 2012). This book is a contribution to expanding this body of knowledge, but these elements need to be consistently evidenced in some form in order for young people's participation to be shared, improved and embedded in ways that enable real change in cultures and practice. But this need for evidence must be integrated into existing systems and processes as much as possible to avoid becoming too onerous, and also be part of a wider learning culture which involves young people alongside professionals in the research and evaluation process (Brady, 2017). Partnership with researchers and young people, as in Chapters 3, 6 and 7 offer an opportunity to develop and co-produce the knowledge base in this area, as well as to develop participative practice.

One size doesn't fit all: the need for flexibility

Who is involved?

As discussed in the Introduction there are disparities in the characteristics of children and young people likely to participate in health services and uncertainty about how to increase the diversity of children and young people involved (Ocloo and Matthews, 2016; Alderson et al, 2019). Less often heard or marginalised young people may need support and encouragement to be involved in strategic participation, but suggesting that they need to be 'empowered' to have a voice in adult decision-making processes and require specific knowledge, experience and skills implies that young people need to adapt to adult ways of working rather than adult professionals developing more collaborative and authentic participatory practice (Brady, 2017). Young contributors to this book have written powerfully about the benefits of participation for their peers, as well as personal benefits including being able to use their lived experiences to create positive change. However, doing this safely requires building trust and personal relationships with the adults supporting participation, as well as being flexible and aware that some young people involved in participation may not want to be credited if that involves highlighting their use of particular services. It is also important to remember that not all young people want or are able to be involved. Inclusive participation requires providing opportunities for any young people who want to be involved to do so in ways that work for them, but acknowledging that if, when and how they are able to be involved is ultimately a matter of individual choice. Young people have a right to be involved in matters that affect them, but they also have a right not to be involved (Brady, 2017).

Structures and processes of participation

The dominant structures for strategic participation in the NHS are formal groups such as youth forums and advisory groups (Crowley, 2015). When approached reflectively and critically these can be a very useful way to involve young people both nationally and locally, as discussed in Chapter 3. Young people's advisory groups are also a popular way to involve young people in health research in order to inform policy and practice (for example Chapters 6 and 7). But structures of participation have implications for how young people are involved, and who is and is not included as well as for adult-child power relations. Considering the processes by which young people are involved is as important as the structures of participation, particularly when seeking to embed more inclusive and socially just participatory practice (Todd, 2012). A collaborative approach in which participation is seen as a context-specific, sustainable and embedded process involving emergent learning, rather than a stand-alone, one-off project, requires clear aims, outcomes and underpinning structures (Davis and Smith, 2012). Structures and outcome measures also need to be 'live' and flexible enough to adapt to the changing needs of services and young people (Brady, 2017). For example in Chapter 4 Sparrow and Linney discuss how the Royal College of Paediatrics and Child Health moved away from a young people's panel to a 'voice diversity' model which incorporates a variety of methods to involve diverse children and young people in ways that work for them, and also enable healthcare services to involve diverse groups of young people and/or those with specific lived experience. In Chapter 6, Percy-Smith et al outline a move away from:

...project-based opportunities for involving children through, for example, young people's advisory groups or one-off consultations, instead focus[ing] ... on developing a wider spectrum of opportunities for participation in more direct and active ways in order to develop and sustain involvement.

Many participation structures are based on the idea of young people having ongoing involvement with an organisation or service, for example as a member of a youth forum or advisory group, and indeed many of the examples discussed in this book are co-authored by young people who have had such roles. But young people using NHS services may not have ongoing involvement with that service or identify with the wider organisation of which the service is a part. As discussed in the Introduction different forms and levels of participation may be appropriate in different circumstances and for different young people. In Chapter 5 Starbuck et al explore how opportunities for participation are 'particularly important for [young people] who face stigma, discrimination and barriers to accessing services'. As with other contributors to the book they highlight the key to good practice in engaging young people whose voices are less often heard as being 'flexibility and willingness to take the perspective of the young people', as well as the importance of building trust and partnerships with specialist services and the voluntary sector discussed elsewhere.

A rights-based framework

Gibson et al (2012) argue for an emancipatory framework for public involvement (participation) in health and social care 'which incorporates cultural, political and social dimensions of a diverse and unequal sector and society' in order to empower, capacitate and support people to 'hold the NHS to account' (p 535). Although this framework does not presume to address all of these issues, it seeks to address criticisms of other models as not having a sufficient emphasis on impact (Tisdall et al, 2014) or challenging adult-child power relations (Percy-Smith, 2016). Figure 10.1 is a synthesis of the key elements which emerged from the research which underpins this book (Brady, 2017), drawing also on the learning from Chapters 1 to 9.

Children and young people are at the centre of the model because of the centrality of children's rights to this book, as well as the importance of developing authentic participation in young person-centred ways and in collaboration with young people and in ways that work for them. The key point here is that the focus of embedding participation is on starting with the young people who are, or could potentially be, involved. But at the same time their participation is bounded by 'scope'.

Scope involves defining the services and systems in which that participation takes place, the boundaries within which young people's participation will be embedded. This may include one or more services, projects or organisations as well as young people and families, services, a wider organisation, commissioning and regulatory bodies and the NHS. It may also include families, carers and support services. What might enable or limit young

Figure 10.1: A framework for embedding young people's participation

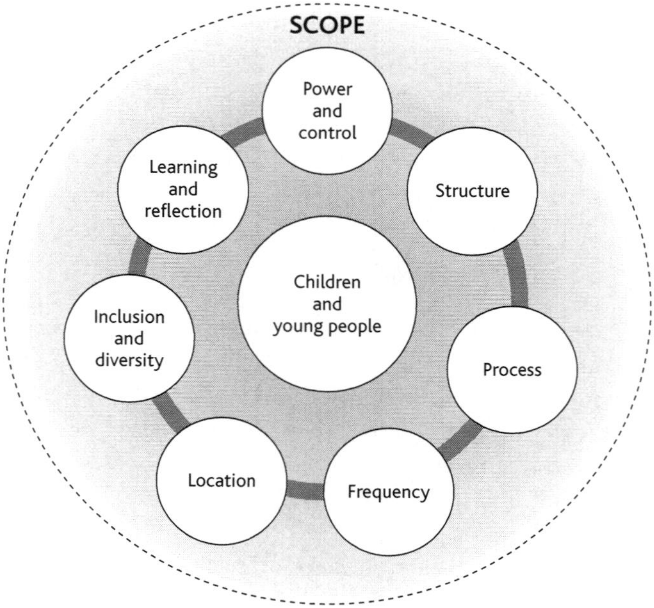

Source: Brady (2017); Brady and Graham (2019)

people's involvement in a service, organisation or programme? What are the policies and processes of the organisation and systems in which participation takes place? What other factors might enable or limit the forms that participation can take and who can be involved?

Within the scope there are a series of interconnected dimensions, set out in Table 10.1, all of which play a part in determining both what young people will participate in and how they will participate.

For participation to be embedded in healthcare practice Brady (2017) found that there needed to be an understanding of all these different elements. A second stage is to identify the systems

Table 10.1: Framework dimensions

Dimension	Key questions to consider
Structure	How can young people be involved? Individually (for example, one-to-one), in a group or both? Is this at a service, organisational or national level?
Process	What level and types of participation are, or could young people be involved in?
	What are the links between young people having a say in their own care (for example, patient experience, shared decision-making) and strategic (for example, participation in policy, service development and delivery and evaluation)?
Frequency	How often does participation happen? Is it a one-off, does it happen at key points/intermittently or is it ongoing?
	How will this work best for the service/organisation/project and for young people?
Location	Does participation take place in fixed or varied locations?
	Does activity take place online or in a physical location?
	Do young people come into adult settings or do adults go to young people?
	Within this also consider whether participation involves going to pre-existing groups or other forums or establishing new ones, or a combination of both.
Inclusion and diversity	Who needs to be included for the participation to be meaningful and relevant to the service, organisation or project?
	Who is and is not currently or potentially included in participation? What would enable them to be included? What might limit their participation, and can this be addressed?

(continued)

Table 10.1: Framework dimensions (continued)

Dimension	Key questions to consider
Power and control	Consider in relation to all of the aforementioned points:
	What say do young people have in what they are participating in, and how, when and where they participate? (structures and systems)
	Who decides what is done with the outputs of participation?
	Who evaluates participation and decides what the success measures are?
Learning and reflection	How will impact and learning from the participation process be evaluated, and by whom?

Source: Based on Brady (2017) and Brady and Graham (2019)

and structures needed to implement the ideas identified through working with the framework in relation to staffing, expertise and champions; evaluation, evidence and impact; reward and recognition for young people involved; training for young people and adults; and what funding and other resources would be needed (Brady, 2017).

This framework is intended as a tool which can be used in both the planning and evaluation of participation. It has been used with organisations thinking about how they can best involve children and young people in their work, and with others who wanted to refine and improve their participation practice by looking at these dimensions in terms of 'where we are now' and 'where we would like to be'. As discussed earlier, different levels and types of participation will be appropriate and valid for different young people, the nature of the specific service, organisation or project and the available resources. Rather than presenting one approach or level of participation as 'better' than another, the intention is to prompt reflection on how to do this in ways that are meaningful, effective and inclusive.

Conclusions

As Kath Evans, who has been at the forefront of promoting children young people's participation in UK healthcare for many years, says in the Foreword to this book:

> participation and meaningful co-production not only
> benefit health services ... [but also] the children and
> young people who engage in the process ... The policy
> drivers exist to support this work ... Our challenge
> is to bring these to life with the children and young
> people who are current and future users of services.

Considering the processes of participation, as well as the structures such as youth forums or other approaches, enables us to consider the relationships between clinical responsibilities and young people's participation and protection rights. This book has explored ideas of young people as change agents and active citizens and presented examples of collaborative and young person-centred participation in shared decision-making, national projects and programmes, collaborative research and young people-led participation. These examples, and the framework presented earlier, provide a means to consider how children's rights and inclusive approaches can be at the heart of young people's participation in healthcare, rather than being a top-down, 'tick box' exercise. Considering *how* young people are involved, and *who* is involved, as well as *what* they are involved in has implications for who is included and excluded from participation opportunities, and for adult-child power relations.

For young people's participation to be truly embedded in health services it needs to clearly be embedded in both national and local policy and practice, backed by resources and linked to outcome measures. In the midst of ongoing national and global political change and the ongoing impacts of the COVID-19 pandemic embedding participation, which is meaningful, sustainable and inclusive in health services requires critical reflection and shared learning as well as an understanding of the wider systems and structures which can facilitate or present barriers to participative practice. As discussed in the Introduction and earlier in this chapter, there is a need for more robust research which maps and evaluates different approaches to involving young people in health services at national and local levels. Related to this and the issues of power and control which run through this book, there is considerable scope for research on developing and learning from models of participation in healthcare which do more to share power, for example considering shared action, co-production and young people-led initiatives. To end as we began, with young people's voices: Ainsworth et al provide a manifesto for this at the end of Chapter 9:

> [young people-led health and wellbeing initiatives are] ... one of the only ways that we are truly going to see a change that benefits young people. Their voice matters, and it is their voice for whom the rest of us must support ... We want radical change, and we want it now. We want the focus to be on collaboration and breaking down barriers, which can be achieved when we stop doing things the way that they've always been done and start stepping out into the unknown.

References

Alderson, H., Brown, R., Smart, D., Lingam, R. and Dovey-Pearce, G. (2019) 'You've come to children that are in care and given us the opportunity to get our voices heard': The journey of looked after children and researchers in developing a patient and public involvement group. *Health Expectations*, 22 (4), pp 657–65.

AYPH (2019) *What's in the new NHS Long Term Plan that is directly relevant to young people's health?* London: Association for Young People's Health. Available from: www.youngpeopleshealth.org.uk/whats-in-the-new-nhs-long-term-plan-that-is-directly-relevant-to-young-peoples-health

Brady, L.M. (2017) *Rhetoric to reality: An inquiry into embedding young people's participation in health services and research.* PhD thesis, University of the West of England. Available from: http://eprints.uwe.ac.uk/29885

Brady, L.M. and Graham, B. (2019) *Social Research with Children and Young People: A Practical Guide.* Bristol: Policy Press.

Brady, L.M., Hathway, F. and Roberts, R. (2018) A case study of children's participation in health policy and practice. In P. Beresford and S. Carr (eds.) (2018) *Social Policy First Hand.* Bristol: Policy Press, pp 62–73.

Coyne, I. (2008) Children's participation in consultations and decision-making at health service level: a review of the literature. *International Journal of Nursing Studies*, 45 (11), pp 1682–9.

Cree, V.E., Kay, H. and Tisdall, K. (2002) Research with children: Sharing the dilemmas. *Child and Family Social Work*, 7 (1), pp 47–56.

Crowley, A. (2015) Is anyone listening? The impact of children's participation on public policy. *International Journal of Children's Rights*, 23 (3), pp 602–21.

Davis, J.M. (2011) Participation, disabled young people and integrated children's services. In J.M. Davis *Integrated Children's Services*. London: SAGE, pp 79–90.

Davis, J.M. and Smith, M. (2012) Participation and multi-professional working. In J.M. Davis and M. Smith *Working in Multi-Professional Contexts*. London: SAGE, pp 36–137.

Evans, K. (2016) Listen and learn. *Journal of Family Health*, 26 (3), pp 44–6.

Gibson, A., Britten, N. and Lynch, J. (2012) Theoretical directions for an emancipatory concept of patient and public involvement. *Health*, 16 (5), pp 531–47.

Hargreaves, D.S., Lemer, C., Ewing, C., Cornish, J., Baker, T., Toma, K., Saxena, S., McCulloch, B., McFarlane, L., Welch, J., Sparrow, E., Kossarova, L., Lumsden, D.E., Ronny, C. and Cheung, L.H. (2019) Measuring and improving the quality of NHS care for children and young people. *Archives of Disease in Childhood*, 104, pp 618–21.

Hood, S., Kelley, P. and Berry, M. (1996) Children as research subjects: A risky enterprise. *Children & Society*, 10 (2), pp 117–28.

Hudson, B. (2018) Citizen accountability in the 'New NHS' in England. *Critical Social Policy*, 38 (2), pp 418–27.

Kirby, P., Lanyon, C., Cronin, K. and Sinclair, R. (2003) *Building a culture of participation: Involving children and young people in policy, service planning, delivery and evaluation*. (Report and Handbook) London: DfES.

NHS England (2017) *Patient and public participation policy*. Available from: www.england.nhs.uk/publication/patient-and-public-participation-policy/

NHS England (2019) *The NHS Long Term Plan.* Available from: www.longtermplan.nhs.uk/publication/nhs-long-term-plan/

Ocloo, J. and Matthews, R. (2016) From tokenism to empowerment: Progressing patient and public involvement in healthcare improvement. *BMJ Quality and Safety*, 25 (8), pp 1–7.

Participation Works (2010) *Listen and change: A guide to children and young people's participation rights.* 2nd edition. London: Participation Works. Available from: www.crae.org.uk/publications-resources/listen-and-change-a-guide-to-children-and-young-peoples-participation-rights-(2nd-ed)/

Percy-Smith, B. (2016) Negotiating active citizenship: Young people's participation in everyday spaces. In K.P. Kallio, S. Mills and T. Skelton (eds.) (2016) *Politics, Citizenship and Rights.* Singapore: Springer Singapore, pp 401–22.

RCPCH (2019) *What do young people want in the NHS Long Term Plan?* London: Royal College of Paediatrics and Child Health. Available from: www.rcpch.ac.uk/resources/what-do-young-people-want-nhs-long-term-plan

Redsell, S. and Hastings, A. (2010) *Listening to Children and Young People in Healthcare Consultations.* Oxon: Radcliffe.

Tisdall, E.K.M., Hinton, R., Gadda, A.M. and Butler, U.M. (2014) Introduction: Children and young people's participation in collective decision-making. In E.K.M. Tisdall, A.M. Gadda and U.M. Butler (eds.) (2014) *Children and Young People's Participation and its Transformative Potential: Learning from across Countries.* London: Palgrave Macmillan, pp 1–21.

Todd, L. (2012) Critical dialogue, critical methodology: Bridging the research gap to young people's participation in evaluating children's services. *Children's Geographies*, 10 (2), pp 187–200.

Viner, R.M., Ashe, M., Cummins, L., Donnellan, M., Friedemann Smith, C., Kitsell, J., Lok, W., Oyinlola, J., Pall, K., Rossiter, A., Stiller, C., de Sa, J. and Pritchard-Jones, K. (2017) *State of child health: Report 2017.* Royal College of Paediatrics and Child Health. Available from: www.rcpch.ac.uk/resources/state-child-health-2017-full-report

Wright, P., Turner, C., Clay, D. and Mills, H. (2006) *Involving children and young people in developing social care.* Participation Practice Guide 06, London: SCIE. Available from: www.scie.org.uk/publications/guides/guide11/

Index

Note: EoF is used as an abbreviation for 'end-of-life'.